SpOil Your Pet

A Practical Guide to Using
Essential Oils in Dogs and Cats
Second Edition

Mia K. Frezzo, DVM
Jan C. Jeremias, MSc.

©2019 by Jan C. Jeremias, MSc and Mia K. Frezzo, DVM

ISBN: 978-1-951044-02-2

Graphic Design: Samantha Kish

Disclaimer: Mia K. Frezzo, DVM and Jan C. Jeremias MSc. are providing this information for informational purposes only; it has not been evaluated by the Food and Drug Administration. Always follow the usage directions given on product labels. The information in this book does not replace veterinary medical advice. Please consult your healthcare practitioner for advice and care. This book is not intended to be used to diagnose, treat, cure or prevent disease.

Printed and Bound in the U.S.A.

Welcome

Dedications

I am forever grateful to Jan for changing my life by introducing me to essential oils.

I dedicate this book to my children who inspired me to seek natural, safe and effective remedies for common ailments. Through those positive, empowering experiences, I began to expand my knowledge and use of essential oils for my veterinary patients. I feel proud to incorporate essential oils in my veterinary practice. I am entrusted with the health, well-being and happiness of my patients, and I feel confident achieving those goals using pure essential oils.

- Mia K. Frezzo, DVM

I am grateful to my parents, and to my friends and teachers for their support and love.

I dedicate this book to my dog Kasey who showed me the power of essential oils and a complementary way of healing and wellness. This singular experience ignited a passion in me to incorporate essential oils in my life and to share my enthusiasm for this healing modality with others.

- Jan C. Jeremias, MSc

Mia K. Frezzo, DVM

Dr. Mia Frezzo is a veterinarian, wife and mother of three young children who resides in northern New Jersey. Her passion for veterinary medicine was initiated and fostered by her uncle, also a veterinarian, with whom she worked and studied since the age of 14. She graduated from The Ohio State University College of Veterinary Medicine in 1998 and returned home to New Jersey to practice veterinary medicine. She is the owner and medical director of Animal Hospital of Hasbrouck Heights located in Hasbrouck Heights, New Jersey. Dr. Frezzo proudly participated on the veterinary panel at the 2018 doTerra Global Convention. In April of 2019, Dr. Frezzo was appointed as a charter member of the doTerra International Veterinary Advisory Board. Dr. Frezzo's patients, primarily dogs and cats, benefit greatly from from her holistic and traditional approach with an emphasis on natural health and prevention of illness.

Dr. Frezzo became convinced of the power of essential oils when the oils cured her 2 year old daughter of a chronic respiratory illness, and she no longer had to rely on a nebulizer and daily prescription medications. As Dr. Frezzo became increasingly frustrated with her daughter's lack of progress and dependence on medications, she sought other remedies. She turned to Jan Jeremias for help. They had met at their local yoga studio, and she knew that Jan was a scientist and knowledgeable in using essential oils and natural health care. Jan introduced Dr. Frezzo to the power of pure essential oils. Within just two weeks, her daughter's respiratory signs were fully resolved.

It was this profound experience that changed all of their lives greatly, including Dr. Frezzo's approach to the care of her patients. Since that encounter with essential oils, Dr. Frezzo has shared natural healthcare with family, friends, clients and pets both in the United States and abroad.

This experience with essential oils led to a greater friendship between Jan and Dr. Frezzo, and ultimately, to the first and second editions of this book.

Welcome

Jan C. Jeremias, MSc

Jan C. Jeremias, MSc. is a certified yoga teacher and reflexologist. She received a Bachelor's Degree in Biology from Stern College for Women and a Master's Degree in Immunology of Infectious Diseases and a Diploma in Tropical Medicine from the London School of Hygiene and Tropical Medicine-University of London. Jan worked in clinical infectious disease and cancer research centers at Cornell University Medical College and Mount Sinai Medical School in New Your City for over 20 years and worked for the New York City Department of Health (NYCDOH) for 4 years.

While working for the NYCDOH, Jan was introduced to essential oils to help with her 14 year old dog, Kasey who had Canine Cognitive Disorder or "old dog dementia". At first skeptical about the power and benefits of using essential oils, she soon became convinced when her dog began acting and feeling better and lived to the age of 19. Since then, Jan has completed extensive coursework in aromatherapy and essential oils for animals. Her passion for natural health and her scientific background has allowed her to help and heal people and their pets worldwide as she continues to share essential oils with family, friends, students, and clients.

Working and sharing essential oils with people has introduced Jan to many wonderful people, her two business partners and friends, Lillian Brenwasser and Denise Schwendeman and her co-author, dear friend and colleague, Dr. Mia Frezzo, without whom none of this would have been possible.

Acknowledgements

We would like to acknowledge Emily Wright, Connie and Alan Higley, Carrie and Fred Donegan, Denise Schwendeman and Lillian Brenwasser for their support and guidance during the creation of this book.

TABLE OF CONTENTS

Welcome 6

Guidelines and Specifics on Essential Oil Use 8

    What Are Essential Oils? 8
    Essential Oil Quality 9
    How To Use Essential Oils 10
    "Hot" Oils 12
    No-No's 12
    Essential Oils In Cats 12
    Guidelines For Using Essential Oils 14
    How To Use This Book 18

Ailments, Conditions, and Other Issues 20

Commonly Recommended Essential Oils 252

Recipes 260

References 268

Index 278

WELCOME

Welcome to *SpOIL Your Pet: A Practical Guide to Using Essential Oils in Dogs and Cats*.

We love our pets! They are family members, and they deserve only the best. We strive to give our pets the longest, healthiest lives possible and believe that the key to longevity is prevention of illness and maintenance of good health.

Dogs and cats race through life, entering adolescence at 4–7 months and beginning their golden years at age 7. To put it in perspective, they age an average of 6–10 years for each of our calendar years.

Always, follow your veterinarian's advice regarding protecting your pet from diseases, parasites and conditions prevalent in your area. We recommend a biannual physical examination for all dogs and cats. More frequent veterinary visits may be needed depending on the age of the pet and any particular medical condition(s) it may be facing.

We value annual blood work, even in healthy pets to thoroughly evaluate and discover any illness or concern as early as possible. It is important to focus on maintaining good health and well-being

> *I have felt cats rubbing their faces against mine and touching my cheek with claws carefully sheathed. These things, to me, are expressions of love.*
>
> — James Herriot

Welcome

as well as addressing any specific ailments. Blood tests and other diagnostic testing may be recommended more often for certain conditions. Greater success is achieved when care is initiated early in the course of a disease and when a combination of traditional and complementary veterinary medicine is used.

Prevention of disease or illness is imperative. In addition to regular veterinary visits and annual testing, provide high quality nutrition, supplements such as Omega-3 fatty acids (fish oils) and a probiotic, and use essential oils to support your pet's immune system. Essential oils offer complementary therapy, enhancing other therapies and are best used under the supervision of a veterinarian. In some cases, essential oils may offer complete treatment or cure your pet's condition.

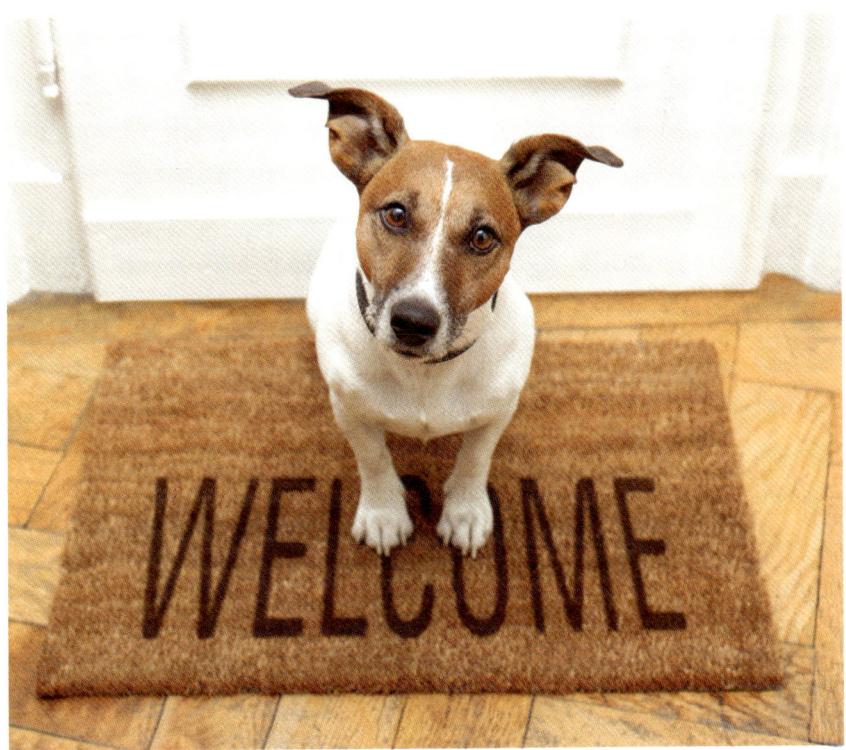

WHAT ARE ESSENTIAL OILS?

Both people and pets can benefit from the power of pure essential oils proven effective for hundreds of ailments. The history of essential oils dates back to ancient times when plants were the first medicines. Essential oils are not new, and modern society is returning to a safer, natural approach to illness and a rediscovery of essential oils.

Each essential oil contains specific benefits to which the body and mind respond. Essential oils are antiseptic and immune system stimulants. They fight viruses, bacteria, fungal organisms, tumors, and more. Essential oils are non-water based phytochemicals made up of volatile aromatic compounds. Although they are fat soluble, pure essential oils do not include fatty lipids or fatty acids, so they are immediately absorbed by the skin.

Essential oils are the volatile aromatic compounds found in the seeds, bark, stems, roots, flowers and other parts of plants. These potent oils, obtained from the steam distillation of plant material, give plants their characteristic aroma. In addition to giving plants their distinctive smells, essential oils are the plant's complex and unique defense system against predators and disease and play a role in its reproductive system.

We consider essential oils a vital tool in the healing of emotional and energetic patterns for both pets and their owners or caretakers. We recommend that you make them a part of your pet's personal healing routine. Essential oils offer total mind, body, spirit and emotional wellness. With each bottle you are holding the pure essence of Mother Nature's healing at a cellular level.

Essential oils effect change by activating the brain's center of memory and emotion, the limbic system, facilitating deep healing of emotional, behavioral, and traumatic patterns. They are easy to use and can be a balancing and uplifting part of your everyday care routine for your pet and for you. This can make an impact at the cellular, spiritual, emotional and energetic levels. They are at work in your cells within minutes of application.

When selected carefully and used properly, essential oils can facilitate the release of old habits, empower change, and restore physical and emotional balance.

Additionally, essential oils offer complementary therapy to traditional medicine, they do not have any side effects and usually do not interact with other medications your pet may be taking. We recommend only the use of certified pure therapeutic grade essential oils that are tested for purity and potency. Always consult your veterinarian when adding anything new to your pet's health care regimen.

ESSENTIAL OIL QUALITY

The majority of commercially produced essential oils are not thoroughly tested for purity, potency and consistency. Thus, the resulting essential oils may contain contaminants and harmful chemicals, including herbicides, pesticides, industrial solvents and phthalates. This potential contamination becomes increasingly important if you plan to apply or diffuse essential oils around your pets. Pets are more sensitive to additives and chemicals than people are.

In addition, poor quality essential oils may contain ingredients that could render the oil ineffective or dangerous. Pure high quality essential oils that contain the appropriate concentration of natural chemicals will ensure that the oils are effective for your pet's needs and that the oils will continue to provide health benefits long term. This is especially important if you are interested in using essential oils preventatively or if your pet is suffering from a chronic ailment.

HOW TO USE ESSENTIAL OILS

We only recommend and refer to 100% pure therapeutic grade essential oils in this book. There are three ways to use 100% pure therapeutic grade essential oils.

They are:

1. Topically, by applying to the fur: Pure essential oils are potent, and a little goes a long way. We recommend diluting essential oils in a carrier oil prior to topical application. Put 1–2 drops of diluted essential oils in your hand, gently rub your hands together, and pet your dog or cat. For cats, allow most of the oil to be absorbed into your hands. Then, pet your cat. Your pet has benefitted from the essential oil if you can smell it on him or her. Petting your dog or cat anywhere on his or her body will be effective as essential oils are readily absorbed into the skin (See Guidelines for Using Essential Oils for dilution instructions). It is more effective to use smaller, more frequent doses of oils than to apply too many drops at one time. Under most circumstances essential oils are applied 2–4 times daily spread out throughout the day and evening. Some pets may appreciate the oils being applied to the abdomen or paws. We feel it is very important to keep the experience of applying essential oils positive for your pet. Most pets do not enjoy having their paws touched or massaged, so we recommend applying the oils to other parts of the body where your pet appreciates touch. For example, the back of the neck, ears, back, abdomen and hind end. When applying essential oils to your dog's ears, be cautious with dogs who have very long ears, such as Hounds or Spaniels in which the ears may transfer essential oils to the eyes (See No No's).

2. Aromatically using a diffuser: A diffuser breaks the essential oil into very small particles, which enter the air and are inhaled. There are two types of diffusers that we recommend. One is a water diffuser that disperses the essential oil into the air with moisture. By using a water diffuser, you can measure the number of drops and observe your pet's response. If your pet seems comfortable, you may opt to add more drops for the next session. A water diffuser allows you to combine several single oils and blends easily. We recommend approximately 6 -8 drops of essential oils per 8 oz. of water.

The other type of diffuser is a nebulizer diffuser, which requires little maintenance or cleaning. The amount of essential oil dispersed into the air is controlled easily with a dial. Start with the intensity setting on low and observe your pet's response.

Pure essential oils should not be heated or burned. These techniques destroy the therapeutic properties of the oil.

When diffusing for the first time, diffuse for 10 minutes and monitor your pet. If your pet shows signs of discomfort such as lethargy, increased breathing rate, panting, salivating, squinting eyes, or any other change that you consider to be adverse or out of the ordinary, simply turn off the diffuser and air out the space by opening windows and doors to let in fresh air. We recommend against enclosing your pet in a room while the diffuser is running, basically sealing your pet into a room without a method of escaping the area if they prefer.

3. Orally: High quality pure essential oils may be ingested. Essential oils may be placed in capsules or in food. For ease of administration, we suggest using prepared essential oil based supplements when possible. If your pet is very small or is unable to swallow medication, we encourage you to recognize that topical and aromatic uses are very effective methods of delivering essential oils to your pets. We do not recommend giving cats essential oils orally.

"HOT" OILS

A few oils produce a warming sensation on the body that may cause sensitivity. Hot oils include Black Pepper, Cassia, Cinnamon, Clove, Lemongrass, Oregano, Peppermint and Thyme. In this book, we do occasionally recommend topical application of Lemongrass, Oregano, and Thyme for specific situations. Use these oils as directed, diluted and with caution. There are other oils that are not considered "Hot" but are considered warming. Examples include, Basil, Ginger, Marjoram, Melaleuca, Pink Pepper and Turmeric (See How to Use Essential Oils).

NO-NO'S

NEVER put essential oils directly in the eyes or ears of your dog or cat. In the event that an essential oil enters the eyes, immediately apply fractionated coconut oil or organic olive oil directly to the eyes. Do NOT rinse or flush the eyes with water as this will not remove the essential oil and will only intensify the uncomfortable and unpleasant sensation. When applying essential oils to your dog's ears, be cautious with dogs who have very long ears, such as Hounds or Spaniels in which the ears may transfer essential oils to the eyes.

ESSENTIAL OILS IN CATS

Cats are a unique species and they differ from dogs and humans in the way they metabolize medications, fragrances and other chemicals. The liver is the primary site for metabolism. Essential oils whether applied topically, inhaled or ingested are absorbed into the bloodstream and processed by the liver. Once in the liver, enzymes convert substances to usable forms. Cats do not possess a particular liver enzyme called UDP-glucuronyltransferase. This is one enzyme responsible for breaking down medications, essential oils and other chemical ingredients. Lacking this enzyme, cats are slower to metabolize certain chemical structures, which may result in higher blood levels and greater sensitivity. Cats are uniquely sensitive to monoterpene hydrocarbons, phenolics and other compounds that contain benzene rings.

Essential oils are not benign substances and must be respected and used with care. Quality, purity, and the dose of essential oil used are critical to safe use of essential oils in all species and especially, cats. Cats are very sensitive to additives. Poor quality essential oils which often contain harmful contaminants are more likely to overwhelm the ability of the cat's liver thereby causing an accumulation of toxic byproducts and signs of toxicity. Signs of toxicity may include incoordination, salivation, disorientation and vomiting.

This does not mean cats cannot benefit from essential oils. Veterinary aromatherapy is not new. By the mid 1800's, scientific studies in Germany and France regarding the medical effects of essential oils on animals and humans were quite advanced. Thanks to positive clinical results, the practice of veterinary aromatherapy was not uncommon in these countries by the middle of the 20th century.

When using essential oils with cats, we recommend beginning with milder oils, and only turning to stronger oils if necessary. We recommend diluting essential oils for topical use, delivering their benefits via diffusion or adding them to the litter box (See Guidelines for Using Essential Oils; and Recipes: Litter Box Power).

GUIDELINES FOR USING ESSENTIAL OILS

- Always use 100% pure therapeutic or medicinal grade essential oils.

- Dilute essential oils in organic oils or lotions. Do not dilute essential oils in chemically laden lotions, soaps or shampoos. We recommend diluting in fractionated coconut oil (FCO). FCO is an odorless, thin oil that is absorbed into the skin readily. FCO allows distribution of an essential oil over a greater portion of the body. Diluting essential oils slows down the absorption of the oil thereby achieving a longer lasting effect, reducing evaporation and decreasing possible sensitivity. For example, when treating pain.

- Dilution Guide for dogs: We suggest diluting to 1%-4% concentration which is 1–7 drops per teaspoon (1 tsp. = 5 ml or 100 drops) of carrier oil. Throughout this book, specific dilution recommendations are made for each ailment or purpose. Please refer to the specific section(s) for guidance.

- Dilution Guide for cats: We suggest diluting even further than for dogs. The dilution rates in the instructions in each section are approximately 0.5%-2% concentration or less. Throughout this book, specific dilution recommendations are made for each ailment or purpose. Please refer to the specific section(s) for guidance.

- Pure essential oils do not stain clothing or bedding. We suggest diluting in a carrier oil prior to applying essential oils to your pets. Please be cautious as carrier oils may stain fabrics, rugs or upholstery. Take care when using pure essential oils as they may damage wood finishes or surfaces.

Guidelines and Specifics on Essential Oil Use

- Remember essential oils are very concentrated. It is best to apply small amounts more frequently than a lot of oil all at once.

- Epileptic and seizure-prone dogs and cats are of special concern. It is believed that certain oils: Basil, Camphor, Eucalyptus, Fennel, Hyssop, Nutmeg, Rosemary, Sage, Tarragon and Wintergreen are not recommended for use in animals with this condition. The reason is that these essential oils may trigger seizures in some people with epilepsy. For this reason, these oils should be used with caution in pets with epilepsy or a history of seizures. We have never experienced seizures in pets in response to using pure therapeutic medical grade essential oils. You may consider substituting Frankincense and Cardamom for Eucalyptus when treating pets with respiratory issues who also have a seizure disorder . Support digestive issues in pets with a seizure disorder by using Cardamom, Lavender and Myrrh instead of blends that contain Fennel and Tarragon. For pets with pain and discomfort, we recommend using Copaiba, Frankincense and Marjoram instead of blends that contain Basil or Camphor.

- Care must be taken with pets who have bleeding disorders, difficulty clotting or who are taking anti-coagulant therapy. If your pet is taking medication for a bleeding and you wish to add essential oils to their health regimen, we suggest include your veterinarian in this decision. In these pets, avoid topical application of Birch, Blue Tansy, Cassia, Cinnamon, Clove, Fennel, Ginger, Oregano, and Wintergreen. Diffusing the above oils is safe (example, Protective Blend which contains Clove and Cinnamon). When treating a pet with a bleeding disorder for an infection, choose Myrrh, Helichrysum, Frankincense or

SpOil Your Pet

Lavender instead of Oregano. Support digestive issues in pets with bleeding disorders using Cardamom, Lavender and Myrrh rather than blends which contains Ginger.

- A pregnant dog or cat is special and therefore care should be taken when using essential oils during pregnancy. These are the guidelines for using essential oils during human pregnancy, we feel that they are also relevant for pregnancy in pets. Caution should be taken when using the follow oils in a pregnant pet: Clove, Cypress, Eucalyptus, Ginger, Marjoram, Peppermint and Oregano. The following oils should only be used in consultation with your veterinarian: Basil, Cassia, Cinnamon Bark, Clary Sage, Lemongrass, Rosemary, Thyme, Turmeric, Vetiver, Wintergreen and White Fir. Use Peppermint essential oil sparingly near the end of pregnancy as it may decrease milk production.

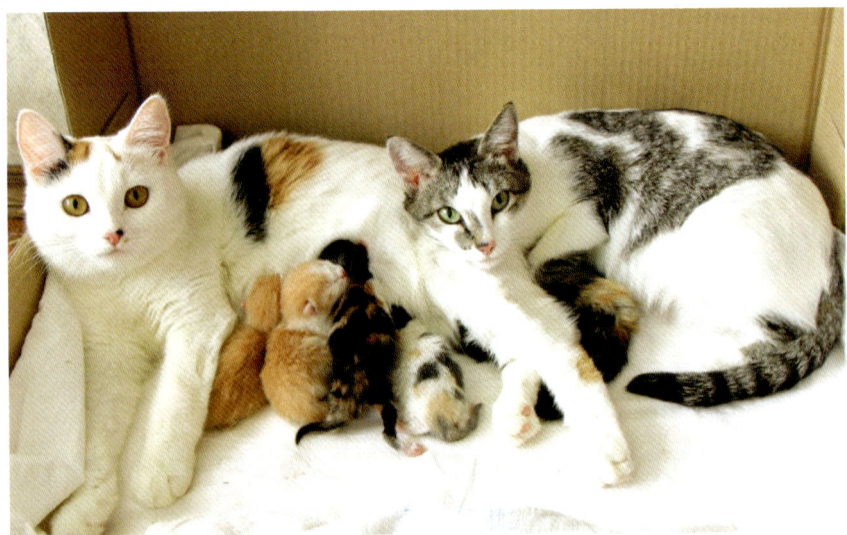

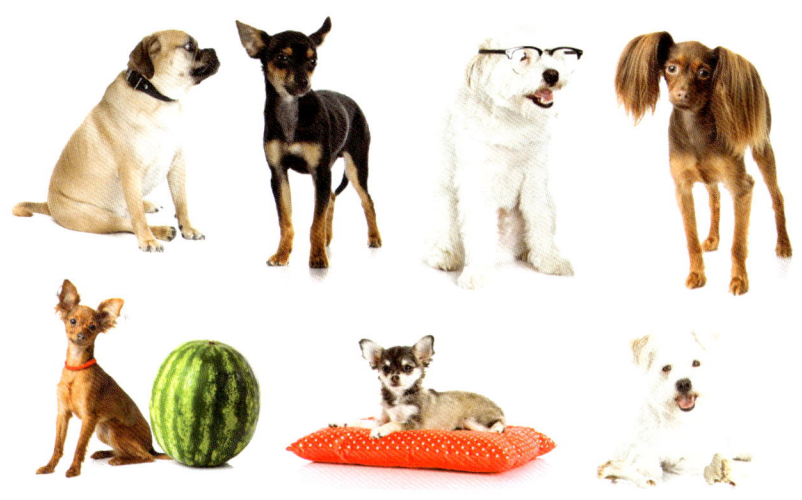

"I hope to make people realize how totally helpless animals are, how dependent on us, trusting as a child must that we will be kind and take care of their needs."

- James Herriot

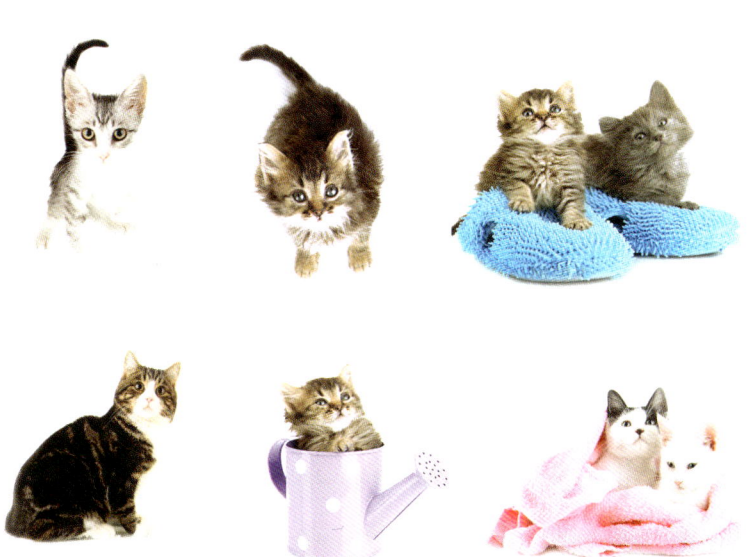

HOW TO USE THIS BOOK

This book is organized to provide dog and cat owners with information about essential oils and how to use them on their dogs and cats. The information is easy to access and gives pet owners practical tools to keep their dogs and cats healthy and to address common medical conditions and ailments using essential oils.

Most essential oils can be used effectively for multiple conditions. In other words, no one oil has just one purpose. In this book, the essential oil(s) we suggest for a particular condition, are our favorites based on scientific research and personal knowledge and experience.

The chapters are as follows: Introduction, Conditions and Ailments, Common Essential Oils, Recipes, and References.

Each section, contains a brief description of a medical ailment or condition, listed in alphabetic order, our recommendations for that condition, and clear instructions for how to use the oils. At the end of each ailment or condition segment is the "What Do I Do section?". Here, are precise guidelines on what to do in this situation for dogs and/or cats. At the end of each ailment or condition are precise guidelines on what to do in this situation for dogs and/or cats.

Guidelines and Specifics on Essential Oil Use

SYMBOLS & COLORS:

Look for these unique icons and colors to indicate information for Dogs, Cats, both Dogs and Cats, and for Emergency and Caution. The icons will help you to quickly and easily locate methods of essential oil use, such as topical application, diffusing, or oral use for a particular situation for your dog or cat.

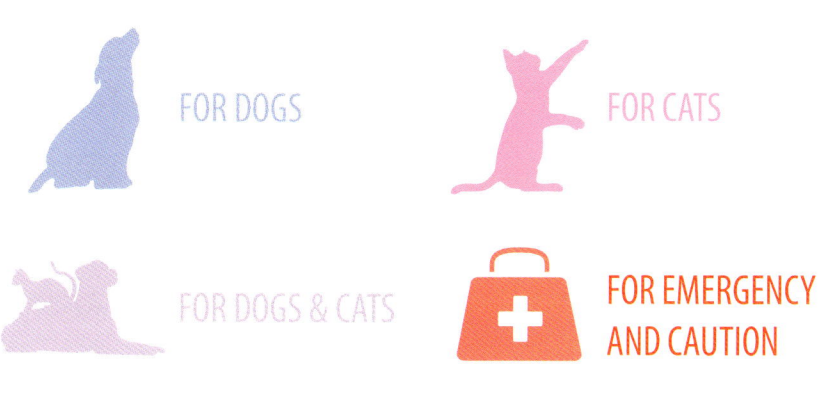

Part of being a pet owner is learning about your individual pet. This book will empower you to help them stay healthy and to take care of their health needs as they arise.

We hope you enjoy this book!

ABSCESSES

An abscess is a pus-filled infected pocket typically located beneath the skin. Most commonly, cats develop abscesses from wounds incurred by other cats. Outdoor cats firmly defend their territory, and males fight over females. A bite or a scratch from a cat deposits tremendous amounts of bacteria beneath the surface of the skin. Dogs more often suffer wounds from fences, playing with other dogs or fighting.

An abscess is generally a raised, warm, painful area of the body. Pets with abscesses are often ill and may develop a fever. They may become lethargic and lose their appetite. If you notice a swelling or painful area of the skin, or your pet is sick, contact your veterinarian immediately.

At home, when you first suspect an abscess, clean the area with a natural cleanser (See Recipes: Gentle Cleanser). Apply warm compresses using a wash cloth soaked in very warm water containing 2–3 drops of Lavender and Myrrh oil for 3–5 minutes 2–4 times daily. Pat the area dry, and apply Healing Salve 2–4 times daily. The abscess will come to a head, open and drain pus and blood. Once the abscess opens and drains, the pet may feel better, but still see your veterinarian. If the abscess does not open, your veterinarian may need to lance, drain, flush the abscess and treat your pet with antibiotics and pain relief.

Essential oils can complement traditional therapies and support the immune system to aid healing. Continue to keep the affected area clean and medicated with ointment (See Healing Salve recipe below).

For dogs, apply a combination of Arborvitae, Lavender, and Myrrh twice daily on and around the wound. Diffuse Protective Blend. Feed your pet a healthy diet supplemented with Omega-3 and probiotics. For cats, apply Lavender, Geranium and Myrrh twice daily. Diffuse

Ailments, Conditions, and Other Issues

Protective Blend. Feed your pet a healthy diet supplemented with Omega-3 and probiotics.

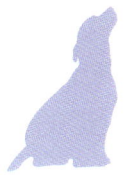

FOR DOGS

Apply 1–2 drops each of Arborvitae, Lavender, and Myrrh diluted in 1 tsp. carrier oil twice daily on and around the wound.

Coat the affected area with Healing Salve twice daily.

Diffuse Protective Blend for 20–30 minutes 2–3 times daily.

Feed your pet a healthy diet supplemented with Omega-3 and probiotics.

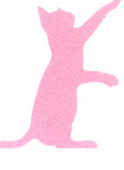

FOR CATS

Apply 1 drop each of Lavender, Geranium and Myrrh diluted in 2 tsp. carrier oil twice daily in and around the wound.

Coat the affected area with Healing Salve twice daily.

Diffuse Protective Blend for 20–30 minutes 2–3 times daily.

Feed your pet a healthy diet supplemented with Omega-3 and probiotics.

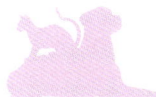

FOR DOGS & CATS

Clean the affected area 1–2 times daily with Gentle Cleanser.

Apply warm compresses using a wash cloth soaked in very warm water containing 1–2 drops each of Lavender and Myrrh for 3–5 minutes 2–4 times daily. Pat the area dry.

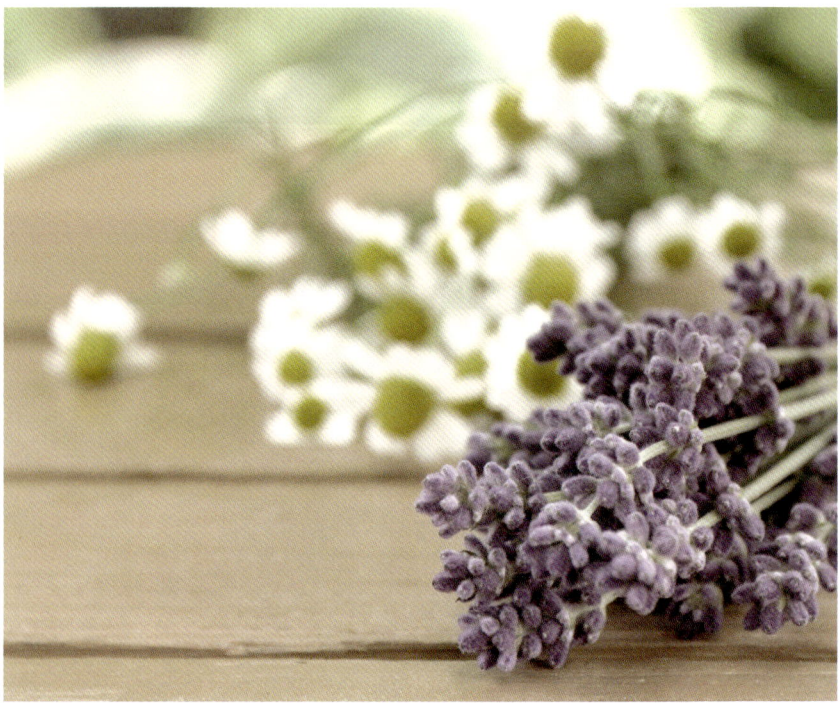
Lavender & Chamomile

Antiseptic Shampoo

Ingredients
10 oz. Water
2 oz. Aloe Vera
1 Tbsp. Castile soap
2 drops Myrrh Essential Oil
2 drops Lavender Essential Oil
2 drops Geranium Essential Oil
2 drops Cleansing Essential Oil Blend
Glass or Plastic Bottle

Instructions
Add essential oils to an empty bottle. Add castile soap, aloe vera juice and water. Shake the bottle well before use. Lather and rinse well.

Ailments, Conditions, and Other Issues

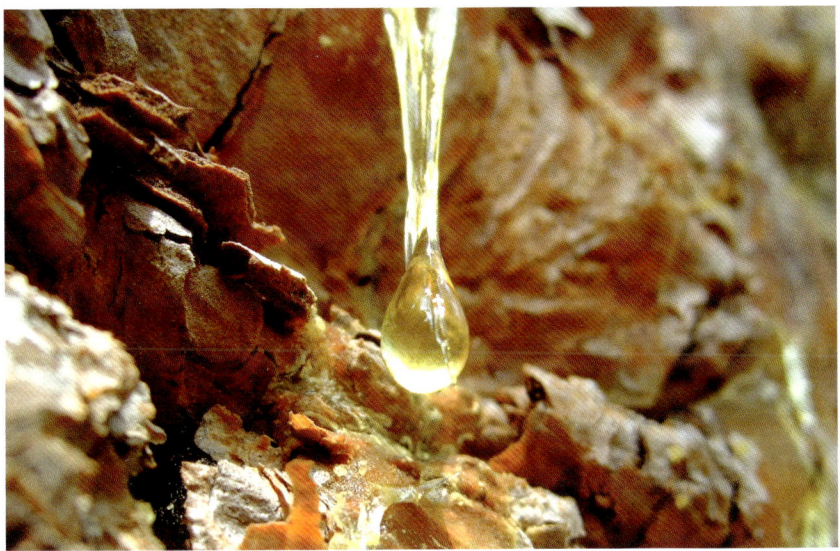

Myrrh

Healing Salve

Ingredients
8 oz. Cold-Pressed Organic Coconut Oil
1 oz. Beeswax
2 drops Vitamin E (optional)
10 drops Lavender Essential Oil
5 drops Myrrh Essential Oil
3 drops Helichrysum Essential Oil
Glass Jars , Tin Containers or Plastic Bottles *

Instructions
Place the coconut oil and beeswax over a double –boiler, and gently warm over low heat until the beeswax melts. Remove from heat and add the essential oils and Vitamin E oil, (if using). Quickly pour the mixture into glass jars, tins, or plastic containers and allow to cool completely. Store salve in a cool location where it will not re-melt and re-solidify. When stored correctly, salve will last for 1–3 years. Yields 8 oz.

ACID REFLUX

Does your pet vomit yellow fluid and foam in the mornings or when he or she has not eaten for an extended period of time? Perhaps, he or she salivates excessively or looks queasy or nauseous. These signs may indicate acid reflux. See your veterinarian for an examination and routine diagnostic testing, such as blood work and x-rays.

Once the diagnosis of acid reflux is confirmed, apply Digestive Blend and give your pet a probiotic supplement to provide healthy digestive bacterial flora, facilitate digestion and support a strong immune system (See Nutrition). Digestive issues can be associated or worsened by stress. Applying or diffusing a calming oil like the Restful Blend may be supportive (See Anxiety, Diarrhea and Vomiting).

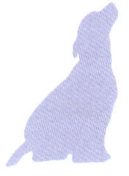

FOR DOGS

Apply 1–2 drops of Digestive Blend diluted in 1 tsp. carrier oil or a pre-diluted roll-on bottle twice daily.

Apply 1 drop Restful Blend diluted in 1 tsp. carrier oil or diffuse for 20–30 minutes twice daily.

Give your pet a probiotic supplement daily.

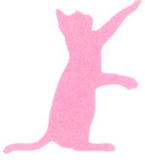

FOR CATS

Apply 1 drop of Digestive Blend in 2 tsp. carrier oil or a pre-diluted roll-on bottle twice daily.

Apply 1 drop Restful Blend diluted in 2 tsp. carrier oil or diffuse for 20–30 minutes twice daily.

Give your pet a probiotic supplement daily.

Ailments, Conditions, and Other Issues

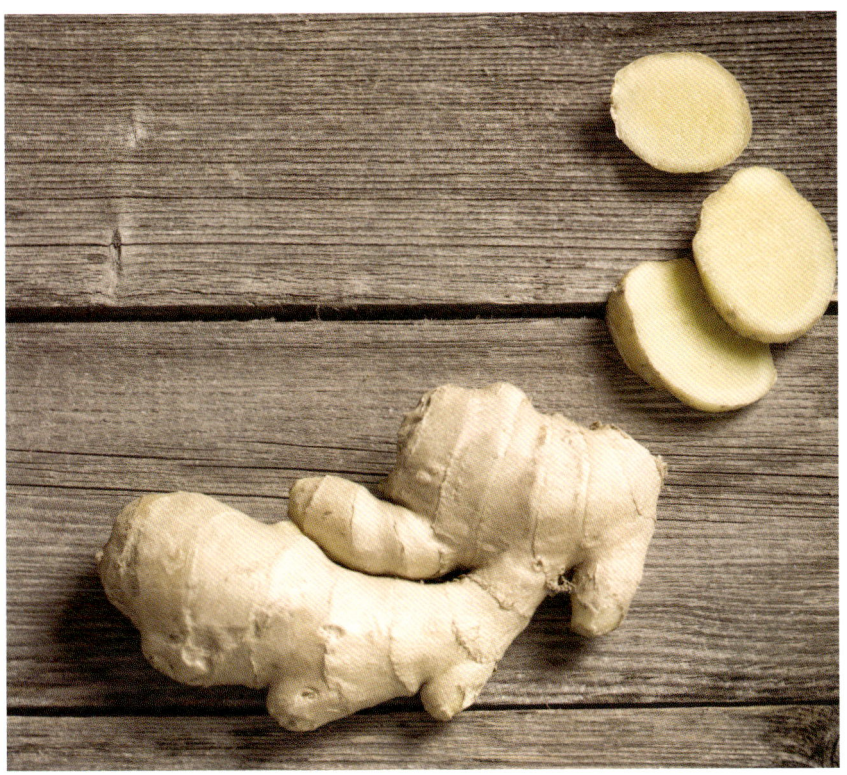
Ginger, found in a digestive blend.

A dog is the only thing on earth that loves you more than you love yourself.

- Josh Billings

ADDISON'S DISEASE

Addison's disease is an endocrine disorder characterized by decreased production of adrenal hormones, particularly cortisol. Both dogs and cats can develop Addison's disease, yet it is more common in dogs. Pets with Addison's disease show severe weakness, anorexia, excessive thirst, vomiting and diarrhea. Addison's disease can be very serious and life-threatening. It is most often caused by an immune-mediated disorder.

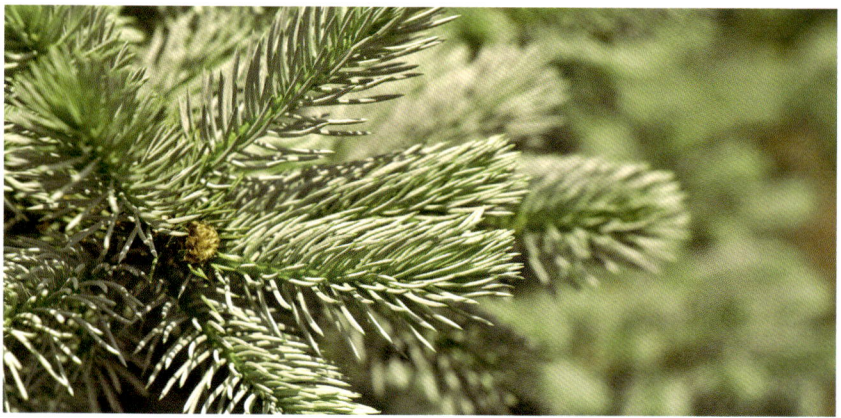

Spruce, found in a grounding blend

If you notice any of the above signs, contact your veterinarian. Addison's disease is usually diagnosed by your veterinarian by blood and urine tests and ultrasonography.

When a pet is stressed, their adrenal glands produce cortisol which helps them deal with the stress. Pets that have Addison's disease cannot make enough cortisol. Therefore, in stressful situations, their symptoms may worsen. Sources of stress vary from dog to dog based on their breed, temperament and personality. Any change in the day-to-day routine, house guests, new baby or new pet is stressful and may worsen signs of Addison's disease or lead to an Addisonian crisis in which signs of weakness, vomiting and diarrhea are very severe (See Anxiety). An Addisonian crisis is an emergency. Call your veterinarian.

Ailments, Conditions, and Other Issues

Support traditional therapy with essential oils. To help with lack of appetite, vomiting and diarrhea, apply Digestive Blend to the abdomen and diffuse Invigorating Blend (See Diarrhea and Vomiting). To assist in cleansing the liver, kidneys, and bladder, apply Detoxification Blend or Geranium (See Organ Support). To support the immune system and maintain overall health, diffuse Protective Blend and apply Copaiba. Apply Frankincense and Grounding Blend twice daily to help balance emotions and the energy of the body. Create a tranquil environment by diffusing Restful Blend or Reassuring Blend. Continue to support overall health by feeding a high quality diet and supplementing with Omega-3 and probiotics.

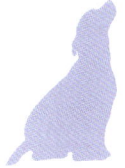

FOR DOGS

Apply 1–2 drops Digestive Blend diluted in 1 tsp. Carrier Oil to the abdomen twice daily.

Apply 1 drop Detoxification Blend or Geranium diluted in 1 tsp. Carrier Oil twice daily.

Apply 1 drop each Frankincense and Grounding Blend diluted in 1 tsp. Carrier Oil twice daily.

Apply 1 drop Copaiba diluted in 1 tsp. Carrier Oil twice daily.

Diffuse Restful Blend or Reassuring Blend for 20–30 minutes 2–3 times daily.

Diffuse Protective Blend for at least 20–30 minutes 2–3 times daily.

Continue to support overall health by feeding a high quality diet and supplementing Omega-3 and probiotics.

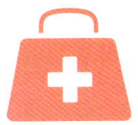

Note: A pet with Addison's disease is delicate and can worsen acutely at any time, especially in response to stress. Contact your veterinarian immediately if you notice lethargy, vomiting, diarrhea or increased thirst in your pet.

AGGRESSIVE BEHAVIOR

Is your dog aggressive toward other dogs or people? Either situation is alarming and can be very scary. Interestingly, the two emotions fear and anxiety are closed linked to aggressive behavior (See Anxiety and Stress). Anger is really misplaced fear. So we may think that our dog is showing aggression out of anger, but much of the time it is fearful or nervous. Signs include, cowering, hiding, barking, growling, showing teeth, lunging, standing rigidly, and raising hair on the neck and back. Dogs have an amazing memory, and traumatic events, abuse and neglect can have a lasting effect. Extensive training, commitment and patience may be necessary to help your dog to overcome these experiences.

Dog-to-human aggression can be unpredictable and dangerous. Dog bites account for a large number of hospital admissions each year and cost insurance companies millions in claims. While most dogs live in harmony with their families, dogs of all breeds and breed mixes have the capacity to bite. Most dogs would rather practice avoidance than bite, but some will resort to biting if they feel threatened or cornered. If the person does not retreat even after the dog has warned him or her, with signs like baring teeth, growling or barking, an incident may ensue.

So what causes this aggressive behavior? Stress and anxiety are leading causes of aggressive behavior. Even though dogs have become valued members of the family, many of them do nothing more than lie on the couch all day. Many dogs instinctually need to work or have a "job". Without a job, dogs are more likely to be bored and suffer from stress and anxiety. Some dogs feel the need to protect their owner, and they take this job very seriously. These dogs do not discern and so may protect us from people we love or people with whom we live. In addition, many dogs receive no formal training. In other cases, owners do not follow through or reinforce training techniques learned from a trainer or in a class. A dog needs ongoing mental stimulation and physical activity.

If your dog is reactive to other dogs, you are far from alone. Tense encounters between dogs are not unusual, as dogs that don't get along with other dogs now seem close to outnumbering those who do. In fact, dog-on-dog aggression is one of the most common behavior problems that owners, breeders, trainers, shelter staff, and rescue volunteers must deal with.

The major reason why dogs become aggressive toward other dogs is that during their puppyhood, dogs are often deprived of adequate socialization with their litter mates and other good-natured dogs. As a result, many pups grow up with poor social skills, unable to "read" other dogs' body language and exchange subtle communication signals with them.

Regular contact with playmates is necessary for dogs to develop social confidence. The current popularity of puppy classes is to provide puppies with a way to experience this vital contact with one another. If puppies miss out on these positive socialization experiences, they are more at risk of developing fear-based provocative behaviors. Because dogs that show aggressive tendencies tend to be kept more isolated than their socially savvy counterparts, their anti-social behavior usually intensifies as they get older.

Pain can easily cause even the nicest dog to bite. Animal control officers, veterinarians, shelter staff members know that an injured dog may not want to be touched and may show signs of aggression in an effort to get people or other animals to leave them alone.

Here are some tips on what to do for an aggressive dog? Dogs that aren't normally aggressive but suddenly develop aggressive behaviors might have an underlying medical problem.

Health problems that may cause aggression include arthritis, hypothyroidism, painful injuries, and neurological problems such as encephalitis, epilepsy, and brain tumors. Talk to your veterinarian to determine whether this is the case with your dog. Treatment or medication may make big improvements in your dog's behavior.

Call in a Professional
If your veterinarian has ruled out a medical problem, it's time to call in a professional dog trainer or animal behaviorist. Because aggression is such a serious problem, you shouldn't attempt to fix it on your own. A professional can help you figure out what's causing your dog's aggression and create a plan to manage it.

An animal professional may recommend training classes, private sessions, exercise, and mental stimulation. Essential oils can enhance your work with a dog trainer or animal behaviorist. Using oils that instill focus and decrease fear and anger will help. Essential oils effect change by activating the brain's center of memory and emotion, the limbic system, facilitating deep healing of emotional, behavioral, and traumatic patterns. When selected carefully and used properly, essential oils can facilitate the release of old habits, empower change, and restore physical and emotional balance.

Myrrh, is considered the mother earth oil offering a sense of nurturing and comfort. Copaiba is very calming and cultivates feelings of worthiness, approval, and acceptance. Cypress is the oil of motion and flow and helps stagnant emotions to be processed and to be released. Juniper Berry helps your dog to face it's fears and offers feelings of courage and energetic protection. Historically, Spruce was used by Native American cultures to promote feelings of strength and security. Emotions such as fear, anger and stress are very heavy, weighing down the heart. Rose offers feelings of love and compassion. Emotions are very complex, and the use of essential oils blends can be beneficial. Blends not only contain a number of essential oils that individually may be helpful but the synergy that is created by combining them is even more powerful.

Ailments, Conditions, and Other Issues

A few of our favorite blends are Renewing Blend, Comforting Blend, Focus Blend, Restful Blend and Anti-Aging Blend. Create a calm, caring and supportive environment for your dog by diffusing some of the above oils for several hours daily. Topical application is powerful by strengthening a positive bond between you and your dog. Based on the oil descriptions above, choose the oils that you feel would best support your dog. In addition, an oral supplement of Copaiba offers powerful antioxidants, neurological support and helps to relieve anxiety. Pets may also benefit from an oral softgel preparation of Restful Blend (Restful Blend oil should not be given orally).

Continue to support overall health by feeding a high quality diet and supplementing with Omega-3 and probiotics. The use of probiotics have been found to reduce anxiety in dogs, particularly by reducing the stress hormone cortisol.

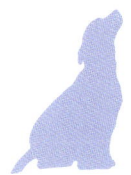

FOR DOGS

Apply 1 drop each of Myrrh, Copaiba and Juniper Berry with 1 drop of either Renewing Blend, Focus Blend, or Anti-Aging Blend in 1 tsp. carrier oil twice daily or more if needed.

Diffuse a combination of Juniper Berry, Cypress with Renewing Blend or Comforting Blend for several hours daily.

Administer 1 Copaiba Softgel (for dogs over 30 lbs.) 1–2 times daily. For smaller dogs, insert a toothpick in the regulator cap of Copaiba and add this amount of oil to the food 1–2 times daily. Administer 1 Restful Blend Softgel (for dogs over 15 lbs.) 1–2 times daily (Restful Blend oil should not be given orally).

Feed your dog a high quality diet supplemented with Omega-3 and probiotics.

ALLERGIES

Allergens and irritants are present everywhere in our environment. Pets may be sensitive to grasses, trees, shrubs, pollen, foods, medications, insect bites, fragrances, grooming products, cleaning products and laundry products. Allergic pets commonly have red, itchy skin especially affecting the face, ears, paws and rectum. Itchy pets will scratch, rub, roll, lick and bite themselves, scoot, and shake their heads.

Addressing seasonal, environmental, or food allergies will help many of the secondary conditions such as ear or skin infections to heal. (See Ear Infections, Fleas, Ticks and Mosquitoes, Nutrition, Skin Infections, Spider Bites). Addressing any underlying causes and feeding a high quality diet is crucial for maintaining overall health. We recommend you have your pet tested for environmental and food allergies, change to stainless steel, glass or ceramic bowls and switch to natural cleaning products.

Allergic pets may scratch so much that they result in skin lesions and open wounds. Skin infections may be treated with an antibacterial/antifungal shampoo (see Soothing Skin Shampoo) followed by applying Lavender and Myrrh or Arborvitae. Lavender contains natural molecules that have antihistaminic, anti-inflammatory and anti-infectious properties. Lavender also helps to

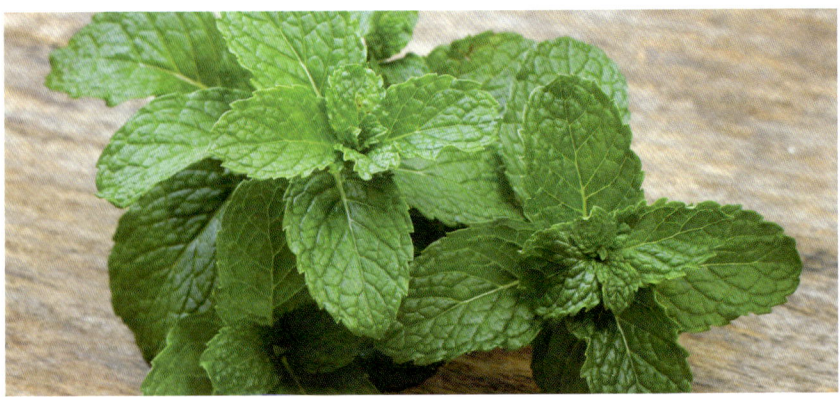

Peppermint

Ailments, Conditions, and Other Issues

repair the skin. Myrrh has been documented to kill many bacteria, viruses, and fungi on contact, so it is excellent as an antiseptic for pets with itchy skin. Arborvitae essential oil has a high content of tropolones, a group of chemical compounds that protect against environmental and seasonal threats, have powerful purifying properties, and promote healthy cell function. Diffusing Protective Blend, Cleansing Blend, or Frankincense is helpful in killing environmental molds and in preventing infection in your home.

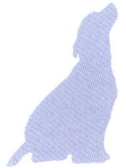

FOR DOGS

Apply 1–2 drops Lavender in 1 tsp. carrier oil or a pre-diluted roll-on bottle 2–3 times daily.

(In an acute case of an allergic reaction, such as an insect bite, 1–2 drops Lavender and Arborvitae in 1 tsp. carrier oil may be safely applied every 2–3 hours, if needed.) (See Spider Bites, Fleas, Ticks and Mosquitoes). Contact your veterinarian.

Apply 1–2 drops each Lavender and Myrrh in 1 tsp. carrier oil twice daily for secondary skin infections (See Cuts and Scrapes).

Combine one drop each of Lavender, Lemon and Peppermint in a empty vegetable capsule or a Seasonal Blend Softgel and administer by mouth 1–2 times daily with food (for dogs 35 pounds or more). For dogs less than 35 pounds, combine 1 drop each Lavender, Lemon and Peppermint in 2 tsp. carrier oil and apply 1–2 times daily.

Diffuse Cleansing Blend, Frankincense or Protective Blend for 20–30 minutes 2–3 times daily.

Bathe with natural Soothing Skin Shampoo.

SpOil Your Pet

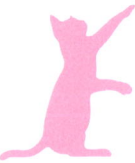

FOR CATS

Apply 1 drop Lavender diluted in 2 tsp. carrier oil or a pre-diluted roll-on bottle 2–3 times daily.

(In an acute case of an allergic reaction, such as an insect bite, 1 drop each Lavender and Arborvitae in 2 tsp. carrier oil may be safely applied every 3–4 hours, if needed.) (See Spider Bites, Fleas, Ticks and Mosquitoes). Contact your veterinarian.

Apply 1–2 drops each Lavender and Myrrh in 2 tsp. carrier oil twice daily for secondary skin infections (See Cuts and Scrapes).

Diffuse Cleansing Blend, Frankincense or Protective Blend for 20–30 minutes 2–3 times daily.

Bathing cats can be challenging. We suggest you find a groomer that specializes in cats and have your groomer use the natural Soothing Skin Shampoo.

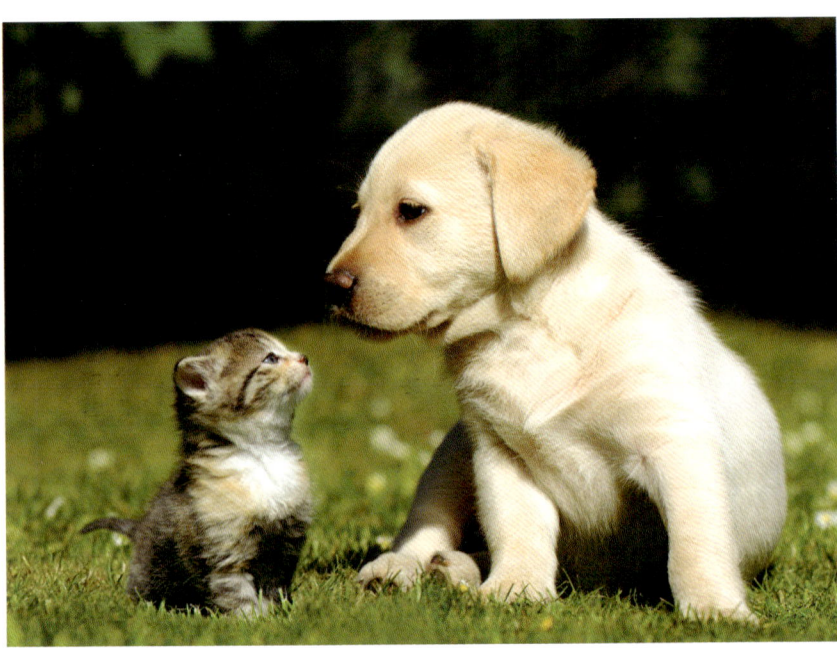

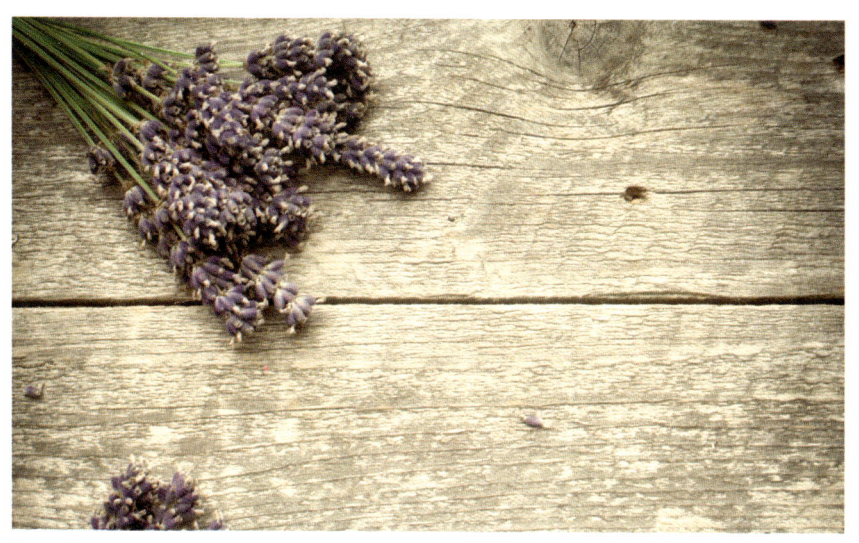

Lavender

Soothing Skin Shampoo

Ingredients
3 oz. Castile soap (available at many health and bulk food stores)
2 oz. Organic unpasteurized, unfiltered Apple Cider Vinegar
1 oz. Vegetable Glycerin
2 oz. Distilled water
3 drops Lavender Essential Oil
3 drops Roman Chamomile Essential Oil
3 drops Myrrh Essential Oil
Optional: *add 1 tsp. ground oatmeal*
Glass or Plastic Bottle*

Instructions
Add essential oils to an empty glass or plastic bottle. Add ground oatmeal (if using). Add the apple cider vinegar, vegetable glycerin, and water to the bottle containing essential oils and oatmeal. Add the castile soap. Shake the bottle well before use.

ANAL GLANDS

The anal glands are located on either side of the rectum at the 4 o'clock and 8 o'clock positions. They should be emptied naturally with each bowel movement and serve as an identification source for other dogs and cats. In cases of diarrhea, constipation, seasonal allergies or food allergies, these glands may become full, painful, infected or abscessed. It is important to identify the root cause, if possible, and address it promptly (see Diarrhea and Vomiting, Nutrition, Allergies).

> *What we have once enjoyed we can never lose. All that we love deeply becomes a part of us."*
>
> *- Helen Keller*

To reduce the pain and inflammation associated with the anal glands, apply homemade Healing Spray and Healing Oil Blend (see recipes). In some cases, the anal glands may need to be expressed by your veterinarian. If your pet is prone to anal gland issues, continue using the natural spray or oil blend. If you can see a red, painful bulge at the side of the rectum or the tissue has ruptured, contact your veterinarian.

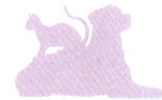

FOR DOGS & CATS

Spray a mixture of Healing Spray and follow with an application of Healing Oil Blend up to 3–4 times daily.

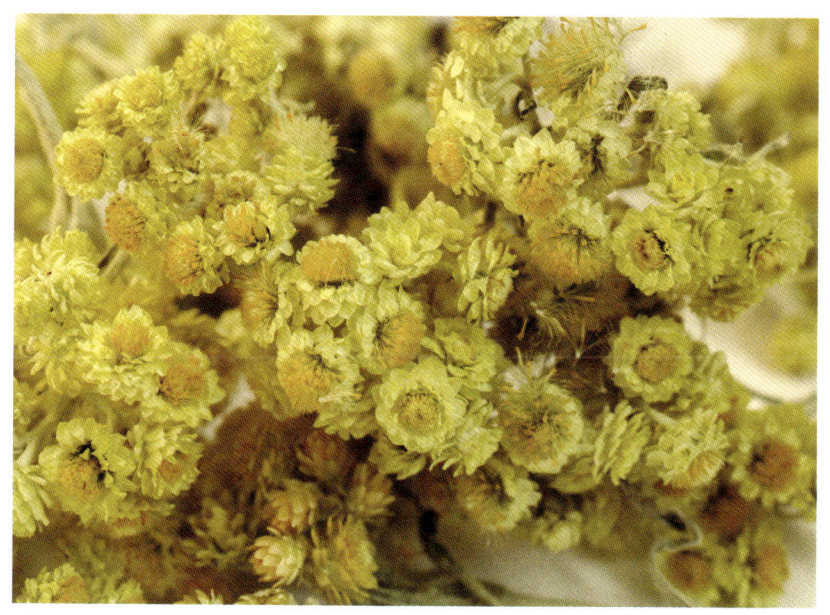

Helichrysum

Healing Spray/Healing Oil Blend

Ingredients
5 drops Frankincense Essential Oil
5 drops Geranium Essential Oil
5 drops Lavender Essential Oil
5 drops Helichrysum Essential Oil
5 drops Myrrh Essential Oil
4 oz. water or Aloe Vera Juice for the spray
    OR
3–4 tsp. carrier oil such as Fractionated Coconut Oil
For dogs only: *If no relief is noted in 24 hours, add 5 drops of Arborvitae to the Healing Spray and Healing Oil Blend.*
4 oz. Glass or Plastic Spray Bottle*

Instructions
Add essential oils to glass or plastic spray bottle. Top with water, Aloe Vera Juice or Carrier Oil. Shake the bottle well before use.
For any condition that persists or worsens, contact your veterinarian.

ANOREXIA AND LOSS OF APPETITE

A pet may refuse to eat or eat less than normal for any number of reasons. In general, one or two days of decreased appetite is not alarming. It is not uncommon and usually insignificant for a pet to turn its nose up at food for a brief period of time, but if this occurs for more than 3 days, it is time to pay attention to the problem and contact your veterinarian.

Many times, there may be a simple explanation such as stress or depression (See Anxiety and Stress, Grief and Loss). In other cases, eating garbage or having a taste of table food can lessen a pet's interest in their own food (See Nutrition). However, a number of more serious medical conditions can interfere with a pet's appetite. If loss of appetite or complete refusal to eat persists for three or more days, contact your veterinarian.

Important: If you suspect that your pet has swallowed a foreign object, string, toy, clothing, coin, chemical or toxin, contact your veterinarian immediately. Pets with a foreign body usually do not eat and are often vomiting.

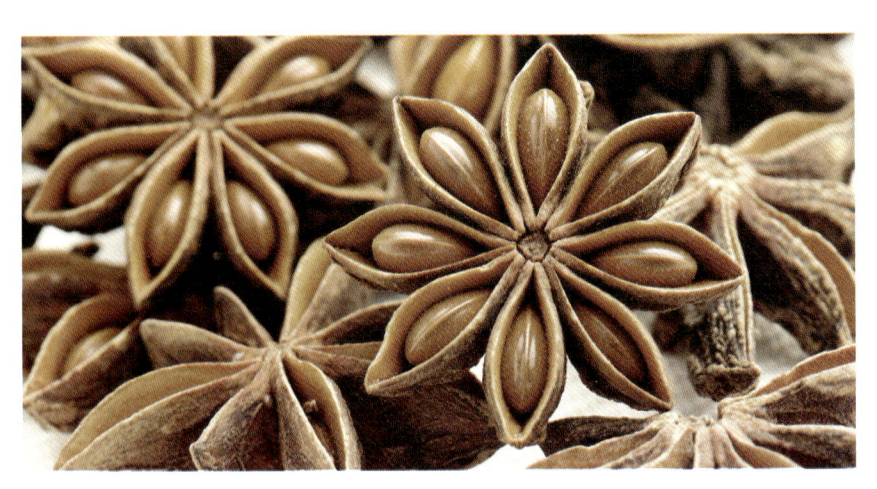

Anise, found in a digestive blend

Ailments, Conditions, and Other Issues

For simple cases of decreased appetite, apply Digestive Blend or Lavender and Myrrh oils. In some cases, when your pet's tummy is sensitive, he or she may prefer that you do not touch the abdomen. Pure essential oils are absorbed into the bloodstream readily, so your pet will still benefit even if you do not apply directly to the area of concern.

Diffuse oils such as Comforting Blend, Bergamot or Cardamom to support positive feelings, uplift emotions, and stimulate the digestive system.

Your veterinarian may recommend a change in diet and recommend a Probiotic supplement. Probiotics are very helpful for digestive conditions and maintenance of overall health. If your pet already takes a probiotic, consider increasing the dose for few days.

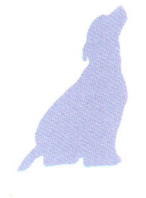

FOR DOGS

Apply 1-2 drops Digestive Blend in 1 tsp. carrier oil or a pre-diluted roll-on bottle 2–3 times daily or 1 drop each Lavender and Myrrh oils in 1 tsp. carrier oil 2–4 times daily, as needed.

Diffuse Comforting Blend, Bergamot or Cardamom essential oil in the general area where your dog eats.

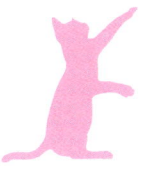

FOR CATS

Apply 1 drop Digestive Blend in 2 tsp. carrier oil or a pre-diluted roll-on bottle 2–3 times daily or 1 drop each Lavender and Myrrh oils in 2 tsp. carrier oil 2–4 times daily, as needed.

Diffuse Comforting Blend, Bergamot or Cardamom essential oil in the general area where your cat eats.

Add Digestive Blend to the litter box as described in Litter Box Power.

ANXIETY AND STRESS

Pets become anxious for a number or reasons. Has your pet ever run under the bed during a thunderstorm, trembled as holiday guests arrive or relentlessly licked at his paw or leg? Does your cat vocalize the entire drive to the veterinary office? These situations are frightening to our pets. Often pets respond by causing damage to the home or themselves, hiding, becoming destructive or having bathroom accidents indoors or outside of the litter box for cats. Additional signs of anxiety in pets include vocalization, pacing, restlessness, panting, and salivation (See Separation Anxiety) .

Another source of anxiety is traveling. Many dogs and cats feel anxious about spending even a short time in the car or traveling via an airplane. Many pets travel to visit family or friends or to stay at boarding kennels while the family vacations or during holidays.

Calm and soothe your pet with essential oils starting a few days prior to the event. Applying or diffusing Lavender and Magnolia, both high in the natural chemical linalool, have been shown to inexpensively, safely and effectively reduce pet anxiety. Lavender combined with other essential oils offers pets greater support. For optimum impact, diffuse Lavender with one of the following: Restful Blend, Comforting Blend, Grounding Blend, Reassuring Blend and/or Frankincense in the home for 30–60 minutes prior to departure. For long drives, a car diffuser is quite handy. An additional option is a pet collar diffuser. Depending on the length of travel and degree of anxiety, some pets may need reapplication of essential oils periodically.

Does your pet have a favorite blanket, bed or toy? Place a few drops of Restful Blend, Comforting blend, Reassuring Blend, Grounding Blend and/or Lavender on the object to comfort your pet. Drip essential oils on the towel or blanket in your cat's carrier. Apply on yourself the same essential oil you are using to calm your pet and act as a human diffuser. The pet will associate the aroma with you and will feel calmer and more secure.

An oral supplement of Copaiba offers powerful antioxidants, neurological support and helps to relieve anxiety. Pets may also benefit from an oral softgel Restful Blend preparation (Restful Blend oil should not be given orally).

Continue to support overall health by feeding a high quality diet and supplementing with omega-3 and probiotics. The use of probiotics have been found to reduce anxiety in dogs, particularly by reducing the stress hormone cortisol.

Add a calming essential oil to the cat's litter box(es) as described in Litter Box Power. If you are boarding your pet with a boarding facility, family member or friend, ask if you may bring a diffuser to calm your pet while you are away.

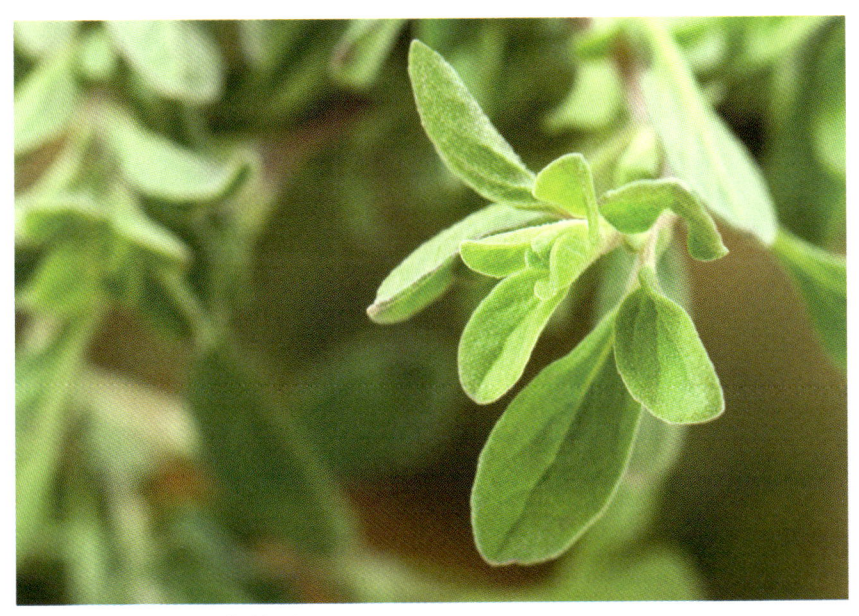

Marjoram, found in a restful blend

SpOil Your Pet

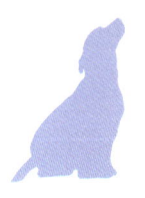

FOR DOGS

Administer 1 Copaiba Softgel (for dogs over 30 lbs) 1–2 times daily. For smaller dogs, insert a toothpick in the regulator cap of Copaiba and add this amount of oil to the food 1–2 times daily. Administer 1 Restful Blend Softgel (for dogs over 15 lbs) 1–2 times daily (Restful Blend oil should not be given orally).

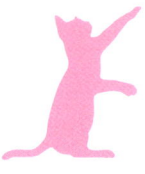

FOR CATS

Add 1 drop each Lavender, Copaiba and Roman Chamomile to 1 cup of baking soda. Allow the mixture to rest overnight in a glass jar. Add 1 tablespoon to the litter box daily (See Recipes: Litter Box Power).

Ailments, Conditions, and Other Issues

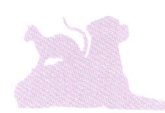

FOR DOGS & CATS

Apply 1 drop Lavender with 1 drop of either Restful Blend, Comforting Blend, Grounding Blend, Reassuring Blend and/or Frankincense diluted in 1 tsp. carrier oil for dogs and 2 tsp. carrier oil for cats as often as hourly to ease signs of anxiety.

Diffuse Lavender with either Restful Blend, Comforting Blend, Grounding Blend, Reassuring Blend or Frankincense prior to a stressful event, before departure and in the car.

Apply 1–2 drops Lavender, Frankincense, Restful Blend, Comforting Blend, Grounding Blend, or Reassuring Blend on your pet's blanket, bed or toy.

Add a Lavender, Frankincense, Restful Blend, Comforting Blend, Grounding Blend, or Reassuring Blend essential oil to the litter box as described in Litter Box Power.

Feed a high quality diet supplemented with omega-3 and probiotics.

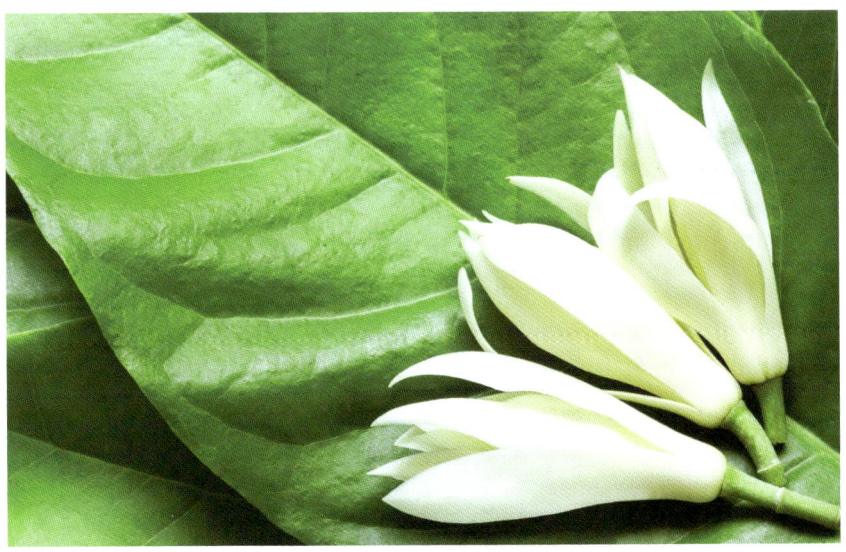

Magnolia

ARTHRITIS

Many pets slow down as they age and exhibit signs of arthritis. Arthritis develops with age, conformational abnormalities such as hip dysplasia, patellar luxations and as a result of joint injuries or surgeries (See Broken Bones, Trauma, Pain, Longevity: A Long and Healthy Life). Certain large dog breeds are genetically predisposed to congenital joint abnormalities, which increases their risk of developing arthritis later in life. In higher risk breeds, it is beneficial to intervene at a young age with protective supplements, maintain a healthy weight and use essential oils.

If your pet is overweight, start with a weight loss program including a proper diet, nutrition and exercise (See Nutrition). Essential Fatty Acids supplements, also known as fish oil or Omega-3, specifically prepared for pets reduces inflammation and supports the immune system. A polyphenol supplement containing extracts from Frankincense Gum Resin, Curcumin (Turmeric), Ginger Root, Green Tea, Pomegranate Fruit, Grape Seed, and Resveratrol and an oral preparation of Copaiba offer powerful relief from soreness and discomfort. Additionally, pet supplements containing chondroitin sulfate, glucosamine and MSM are quite helpful. Supplements and natural alternatives can replace or lessen the necessity for traditional medications in many cases.

Essential oils have been found to reduce pain, inflammation and stiffness. In many cases, topical application of Massage Blend is helpful. This blend not only relieves pain but also helps to repair injured tissue, soothe muscles and enhance blood flow. For greater support and enhanced relief, add Copaiba, Turmeric, Frankincense or Lavender. Turmerones, the main constituent in Turmeric, are among the most powerful naturally-occurring anti-inflammatories.

Ailments, Conditions, and Other Issues

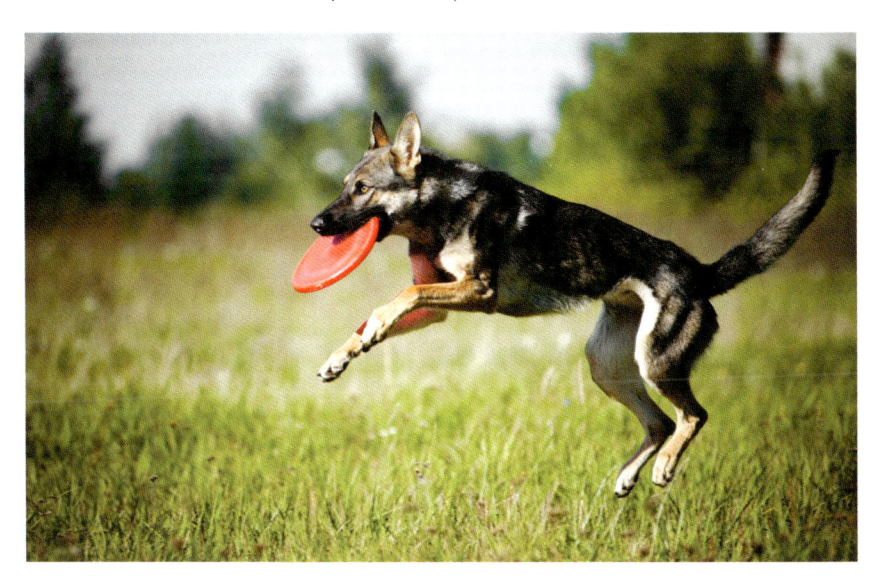

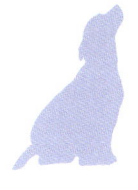

FOR DOGS

Apply 1- 2 drops Massage Blend in 1 tsp. carrier oil 2–4 times daily.

For greater support, add 1 drop of Massage blend and 1 drop of either Copaiba, Turmeric, Frankincense or Lavender in 1 tsp. carrier oil to the palms of your hands, and simply pet your dog. Pet the area of concern or anywhere on your pet's body 2–4 times daily as needed.

Administer 1 Polyphenol Complex (for dogs over 45 lbs) and/or 1 Copaiba Softgel (for dogs over 30 lbs) 1–2 times daily. For smaller dogs, insert a toothpick in the regulator cap of Copaiba and add this amount of oil to the food 1–2 times daily.

Diffuse Copaiba and Ginger for 20–30 minutes 2–3 times daily.

Pure essential oils are absorbed into the bloodstream readily, so your pet will still benefit even if you do not apply directly to the area of concern.

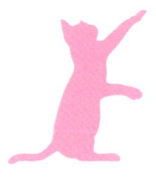

FOR CATS

Dilute 1 drop of Massage Blend in 2 tsp. carrier oil and apply 2–4 times daily.

For greater support, add 1 drop of Massage blend and 1 drop of either Copaiba, Turmeric, Frankincense or Lavender in 2 tsp. carrier oil to the palms of your hands, and simply pet your cat. Pet the area of concern or anywhere on your pet's body 2–4 times daily as needed.

Diffuse Copaiba and Ginger for 20–30 minutes 2–3 times daily.

Pure essential oils are absorbed into the bloodstream readily, so your pet will still benefit even if you do not apply directly to the area of concern.

"Pets have more love and compassion in them than most humans."

- Robert Wagner

Ailments, Conditions, and Other Issues

AUTOIMMUNE DISORDERS

Autoimmune disorders are difficult to understand. Suddenly, and many times, for no apparent reason, the body begins to attack itself. What? It sounds crazy, but it is true. An autoimmune disorder occurs, when the body's immune system targets the pet's own healthy tissue and cells. The cause in many cases is unknown, but in some cases the development of an autoimmune condition has been found to be genetic, following an infection or the administration of some medications. Sometimes the organ of attack is a blood cell type, such as the red blood cells. In other cases, autoimmune disorders may cause skin lesions. Because of the variety of signs and causes of autoimmune disease, bring your pet to your veterinarian whenever you notice unusual changes in appearance or behavior. Some signs are bruises or areas of hemorrhage in the skin and gums, non-healing skin wounds, loss of pigment localized to the eyes, nose and mouth and lethargy. Any of these conditions require diagnostic testing, treatment and monitoring by your veterinarian. Essential oils offer your pet complementary therapy by strengthening the immune system and controlling infection. . Use safe household cleaning and grooming products and support your pet's immune system and healing with a healthy diet, Omega-3 and Probiotic supplements.

For dogs, apply Copaiba, Frankincense, Grounding Blend and Helichrysum daily and diffuse Protective Blend or Frankincense.

"Animals are reliable, many full of love, true in their affections, predictable in their actions, grateful and loyal. Difficult standards for people to live up to."

- Alfred A. Montapert

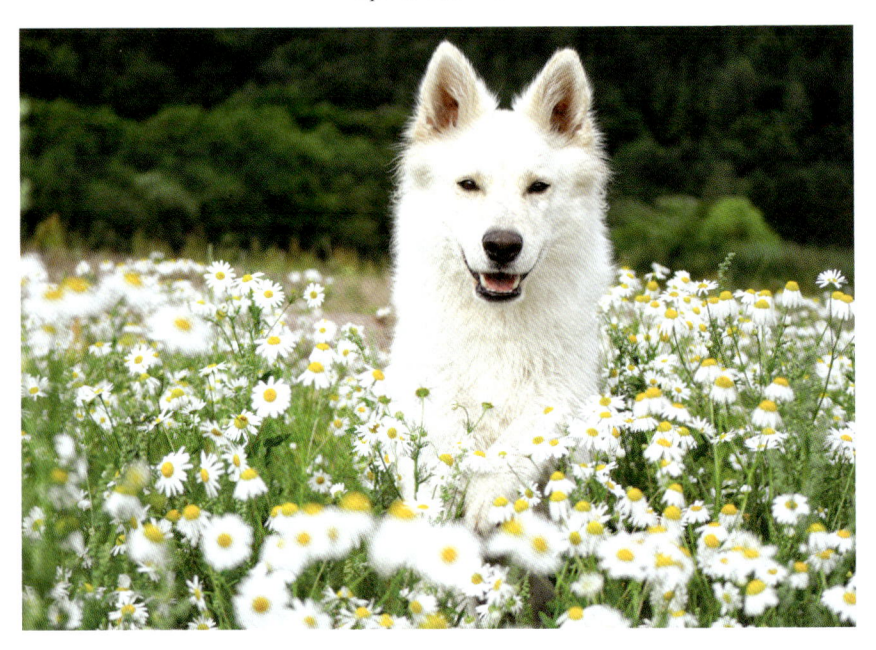

These oils help to heal skin conditions, support the immune system and relieve tension and anxiety. A Cellular Complex, an oral preparation, containing Frankincense, Wild Orange, Litsea, Thyme, Clove, Summer Savory, Niaouli, and Lemongrass essential oils and an oral supplement of Copaiba offers powerful antioxidants, immune system support and helps to relieve discomfort

For cats, apply Copaiba, Helichrysum, Frankincense and Myrrh and diffuse Protective Blend or Frankincense. These oils help to heal skin conditions, support the immune system and relieve tension and anxiety.

Ailments, Conditions, and Other Issues

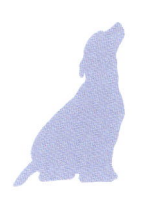

FOR DOGS

Apply 1 drop each of Frankincense, Copaiba, Grounding Blend and Helichrysum in 1 tsp. carrier oil twice daily.

Administer 1 Cellular Complex (for dogs over 50 lbs). For smaller dogs, under 25 lbs administer 1 drop Cellular Compex twice daily with food, for dogs 25–50 lbs administer 1 drop Cellular Complex 4 times daily with food.

Administer 1 Copaiba Softgel (for dogs over 30 lbs) 1–2 times daily. For smaller dogs, insert a toothpick in the regulator cap of Copaiba and add this amount of oil to the food 1–2 times daily.

Diffuse Protective Blend or Frankincense for 20–30 minutes twice daily.

Feed a healthy diet and supplement with Omega-3 and probiotics.

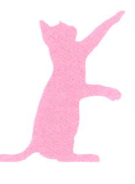

FOR CATS

Apply 1 drop each Frankincense, Copaiba, Helichrysum and Myrrh 2 tsp. carrier oil 1–2 times daily.

Diffuse Protective Blend or Frankincense for 20–30 minutes twice daily.

Feed a healthy diet and supplement with Omega-3 and probiotics.

BARTONELLA (CAT SCRATCH FEVER)

Bartonella or Cat Scratch Fever is a bacterial disease contagious to people and very common among cats. In fact, about 30% of healthy cats are carriers of this disease and show no signs of illness. Bartonella is spread by fleas and ticks (See Fleas, Ticks and Mosquitoes). Dogs rarely become infected with Bartonella.

Bartonella can affect many body systems, so the signs may be varied. Signs of Bartonella include conjunctivitis, sneezing, runny nose, gingivitis, oral ulcers, heart disease, diarrhea, vomiting, fever and dermatitis.

Because Bartonella is so widespread among healthy cats, blood testing is recommended on all cats with or without signs of illness. We suggest testing when a new cat or kitten is acquired to ensure that your pet and family are protected from this contagious disease. Keeping your cat indoors and free of fleas and ticks) will help to protect your cat from contracting Bartonella.

If the test result is positive, Bartonella is treated with antibiotics. Essential oils provide complimentary therapy by helping to support your pet's immune system and assist in his or her recovery from Bartonella and any secondary infections he or she may develop. Essential oils will also help to protect you, your family and anyone who may come into contact with your infected pet until antibiotic therapy is completed.

For rare cases of Bartonella in dogs, apply Arborvitae, Frankincense, Myrrh and Lavender twice daily. For respiratory symptoms, apply or diffuse Frankincense and Respiratory Blend. To support the immune system, diffuse Protective Blend. For cats, apply Arborvitae, Frankincense, Myrrh and Lavender twice daily. For respiratory symptoms, apply or diffuse Frankincense and Respiratory Blend. To support the immune system, diffuse Protective Blend. For additional support, apply Rose, Children's Protective Blend or Copaiba.

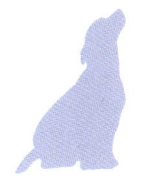

FOR DOGS

Apply 1 drop each Arborvitae, Frankincense, Myrrh and Lavender in 2 tsp. carrier oil 2–3 times daily.

Apply 1–2 drops of Respiratory Blend diluted in 1 tsp. carrier oil or a pre-diluted roll-on bottle twice daily.

Alternate diffusing Protective Blend or Frankincense and Respiratory Blend for 20–30 minutes 2–3 times daily.

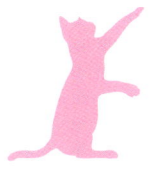

FOR CATS

Apply 1 drop each Arborvitae, Frankincense, Myrrh and Lavender in 2 tsp. carrier oil 2–3 times daily.

Apply 1 drop of Respiratory Blend diluted in 2 tsp. carrier oil or a pre-diluted roll-on bottle twice daily.

Alternate diffusing Protective Blend or Frankincense and Respiratory Blend for 20–30 minutes 2–3 times daily.

Arborvitae

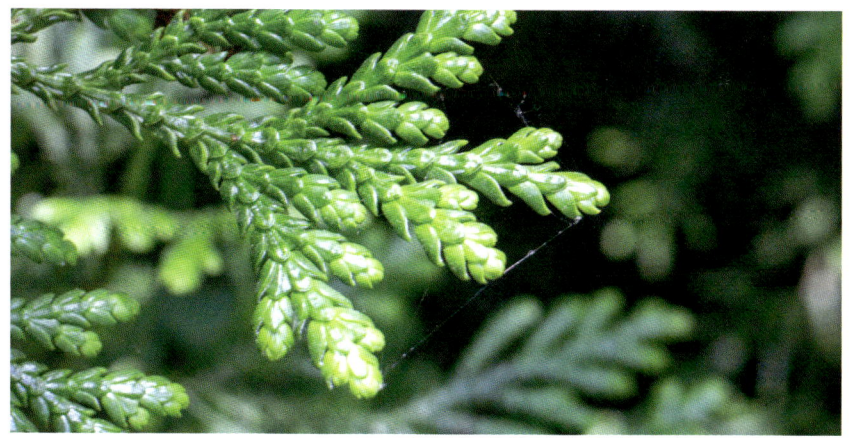

SpOil Your Pet

BROKEN BONES/BONE PAIN

In the event of a broken bone, see your veterinarian immediately. Essential oils can be used to speed healing and reduce inflammation once the fracture is repaired or set.

Essential oils have been found to reduce pain, inflammation and stiffness. In many cases, topical application of Massage Blend is helpful. This blend not only relieves pain but also helps to repair injured tissue, soothe muscles and enhance blood flow. For greater support and enhanced relief, add Siberian Fir, Helichrysum and Copaiba,

Grounding Blend, Lavender and Restful Blend will help to ease anxiety and keep you and your pet calm (See Anxiety and Stress). Healing requires a strong immune system, proper hydration, and good nutrition. Support your pet by providing essential oils, high quality nutrition, a probiotic, and Omega-3 supplements.

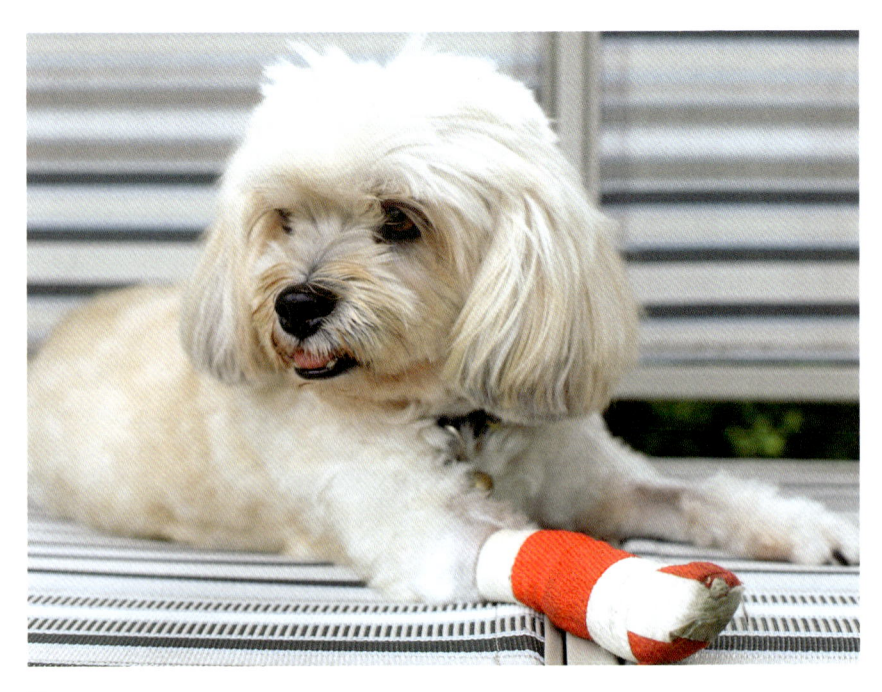

Ailments, Conditions, and Other Issues

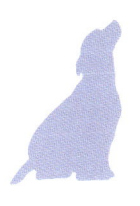

FOR DOGS

Apply 1 drop each Massage Blend, Siberian Fir, and Helichrysum diluted in 2 tsp. carrier oil near the fracture area 2–3 times daily. After 4 weeks, decrease the frequency to 1–2 times daily.

Apply 1–2 drops of Grounding Blend, Lavender or Restful Blend diluted in 1 tsp. carrier oil twice daily.

Diffuse Grounding Blend, Lavender or Restful Blend 20–30 minutes for 2–3 hours

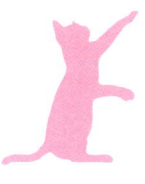

FOR CATS

Apply 1 drop each Massage Blend, Siberian Fir, and Helichrysum diluted in 4 tsp. carrier oil near the fracture area 2–3 times daily. After 4 weeks, decrease the frequency to 1–2 times daily.

Apply 1–2 drops of Grounding Blend, Lavender or Restful Blend diluted in 2 tsp. carrier oil twice daily.

Diffuse Grounding Blend, Lavender or Restful Blend 20–30 minutes for 2–3 hours

BURNS

Pets suffer from two main types of burns: thermal and chemical burns. Thermal burns are heat-related such as touching the stove, lying on the radiator, or overexposure to a heating pad. Chemical burns are from caustic substances such as irritants, acids or bases. Some common causes of chemical burns include car battery acid, cleaning products, bleach, ammonia, denture cleaner, teeth whitening products and pool chlorinating products. Chemicals cause harm through contact, inhalation (breathing in fumes) or ingestion (See Green Cleaning).

In the event of a burn, remove the pet from the source of heat or chemical. Rinse the skin or affected part of his or her body for 10–20 minutes under COOL running water. Cover the affected area with a clean, soft, dry cloth and Seek Veterinary Care Immediately. Do NOT apply butter, ointments or Vaseline to burns. Do NOT apply ice to burns. If you have assistance, apply Lavender or Restful Blend to you and your pet to help keep you both calm.

After your pet has seen your veterinarian, apply Lavender, Frankincense and Healing Salve or Healing Spray daily. Add Frankincense to food (if there are no cats in the home). Alternate diffusing Protective Blend, Lavender, or Restful Blend daily.

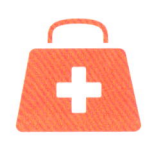

SEEK VETERINARY ATTENTION IMMEDIATELY.

Ailments, Conditions, and Other Issues

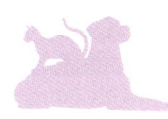

FOR DOGS & CATS

Apply 1–2 drops of Lavender or Restful Blend diluted in 1 tsp. carrier oil for dogs and 2 tsp. carrier oil for cats.(Only if Time Permits).

After your pet has seen your veterinarian:

Apply 1–2 drops each Lavender and Frankincense diluted in 1 tsp. carrier oil for dogs and 2 tsp. carrier oil for cats 2–4 times daily.

Apply Healing Salve or Healing Spray 2–4 times daily.

Add Frankincense to food (if there are no cats in the home). Insert a toothpick in the regulator cap of Frankincense and add this amount of oil to the food 1–2 times daily.

Diffuse Protective Blend for 20–30 minutes at least 2–3 times daily.

Diffuse Lavender or Restful Blend for 20–30 minutes 2–3 times daily.

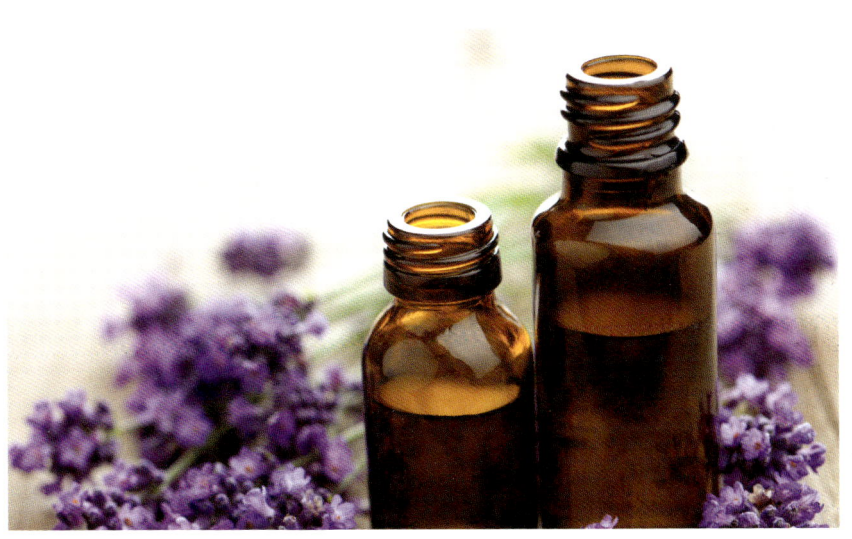

Lavender

Healing Salve

Ingredients
8 oz. Cold-Pressed Organic Coconut Oil
1 oz. Beeswax
2 drops Vitamin E (optional)
10 drops Lavender Essential Oil
5 drops Myrrh Essential Oil
3 drops Helichrysum Essential Oil
Glass Jars , Tin Containers or Plastic Bottle *

Instructions
Place the coconut oil and beeswax over a double –boiler, and gently warm over low heat until the beeswax melts. Remove from heat and add the essential oils and Vitamin E oil, (if using). Quickly pour the mixture into glass jars, tins, or plastic containers and allow to cool completely. Store salve in a cool location where it will not re-melt and re-solidify. When stored correctly, salve will last for 1–3 years. Yields 8 oz.

Healing Spray/Healing Oil Blend

5 drops Frankincense Essential Oil
5 drops Geranium Essential Oil
5 drops Lavender Essential Oil
5 drops Helichrysum Essential Oil
5 drops Myrrh Essential Oil
4 oz. water or Aloe Vera Juice for the spray
   OR
3–4 tsp. carrier oil such as Fractionated Coconut Oil

For dogs only: If no relief is noted in 24 hours, add 5 drops of Arborvitae to the Healing Spray and Healing Oil Blend.
4 oz. Glass or Plastic Spray Bottle*

Instructions
Add essential oils to glass or plastic spray bottle. Top with water, Aloe Vera Juice or Carrier Oil. Shake the bottle well before use.

For any condition that persists or worsens, contact your veterinarian.

Safety Precautions

To prevent chemical burns and poisonings, keep chemicals and cleaning products safely stored away from pets. The following is a list of safety recommendations for the use of chemicals and dangerous substances:

Use chemicals in a well-ventilated area.

Keep chemicals in their original containers which provide the exact ingredients and instructions in case of accidental ingestion or exposure.

Avoid using chemicals.

Do not mix chemicals.

Do not use or store chemicals near food or drinks.

Safely confine your pet away from chemicals while in use.

Wear recommended protection such as gloves or safety goggles when using chemicals.

In the event a chemical is ingested, do not induce vomiting. Call Animal Poison Control* immediately. Consider saving this number in your contact list.

*Animal Poison Control Hotline : 1-800-548-2423
 Animal Poison Helpline: 1-800-213-6680

CANCER

Our pets are living longer lives due to better nutrition, preventative care and advances in medicine. Cancer is often a disease of older pets yet can affect younger pets, too. The prevalence of cancer is rising. Any lump, bump or growth should be evaluated by your veterinarian. Pet owners commonly discover such changes in their pets simply by petting them, brushing and bathing.

Tumors and cancer develop because of an abnormal change in the cell's DNA. Some of these changes may be genetic (due to family history), yet many are random. Several factors have been suggested to play a role in the development of cancer, such as the environment, poor diet and infectious agents. Specifically, household cleaners, chemicals, and cigarette smoke have been attributed to the development of cancer in our pets. Cancers affecting younger pets may be attributed to breed-associated links or viruses such as feline leukemia virus (FeLV) (See Feline Leukemia Virus), feline immunodeficiency virus (FIV) (See Feline Immunodeficiency Virus) and canine papillomavirus.

One of the primary reasons to spay or neuter your pet is to reduce or nearly eliminate the risk of mammary gland cancer in females and testicular cancer in males. When these procedures are performed at a young age (6 months of age and prior to any estrus cycles in females), the risk of these cancers is greatly decreased.

Choosing if and how to treat your pet's cancer is a very personal decision involving several considerations such as type of cancer, prognosis, quality of life, estimated time of survival, and finances. Traditional treatment options for pets include surgery, chemotherapy, and radiation, similar to our own choices for cancer therapy.

Essential oils may be used in conjunction with traditional cancer treatments or instead of aggressive or invasive methods of cancer treatment. Essential oils support your pet's immune system, aid digestion and increase appetite, and improve energy and well-being.

Many essential oils have the capabilities of affecting cancer cells. Frankincense, in particular, has been shown to kill cancer cells in animal laboratory studies. Citrus oils such as Bergamot and other oils such as Pink Pepper and Cardamom contain a natural chemical of particular importance in cancer prevention called d-limonene. This simple compound has been found in nearly 100 studies in animals and in humans to prevent cancer and stop the progression of cancer. It has been shown to be active against several types of tumor cells, including mammary, skin, lung, liver and forestomach in rodents and colon and breast cancer cells in humans. There are numerous essential oils that have been shown to improve health and wellbeing in animals with cancer. They include Frankincense, Sandalwood, Copaiba, Pink Pepper, Geranium, Lavender, Bergamot and Myrrh.

> *"Sometimes you don't need words to feel better; you just need the nearness of your dog."*
>
> — Natalie Lloyd

For dogs, apply the following two combinations alternating weekly: Combination 1 - Frankincense, Sandalwood, Geranium, Lavender and Myrrh and Combination 2 - Frankincense, Cardamom, Copaiba, Pink Pepper and Lavender daily. Apply Grounding Blend for calming and Digestive Blend for digestive upset or to increase appetite. Apply Massage Blend daily for pain relief (See Pain). A Cellular Complex, an oral preparation, containing Frankincense, Wild Orange, Litsea, Thyme, Clove, Summer Savory, Niaouli, and Lemongrass essential oils and an oral supplement of Copaiba offer powerful antioxidants, immune system support and help to relieve discomfort. Diffuse Protective Blend, Frankincense, and Lemon or Grapefruit, to support well-being and purify the air and uplift the mood. Apply Restful Blend to you and your pet, and diffuse Restful Blend to promote a feeling of calm during this stressful time.

For cats, apply Frankincense, Sandalwood, Geranium, Lavender and Myrrh daily. Apply Massage Blend daily for pain relief. Add Digestive Blend and/or Copaiba and Lavender to the litter box as described in Litter Box Power to support healthy digestion, immunity and ease anxiety See Litter Box Power, Anxiety and Stress). Diffuse Protective Blend, Frankincense, and Bergamot, to support well-being and purify the air and uplift the mood. Apply Restful Blend to you and your pet, and diffuse Restful Blend to promote a feeling of calm during this stressful time.

Additional steps you can take if your pet has cancer which are generally good practice include converting to natural cleaners and air fresheners, removing toxins and switching to natural grooming products. Use natural or unscented cat litter, and feed a diet free from preservatives and chemicals. Support your pet by feeding a high quality diet and supplement Omega-3 and probiotics.

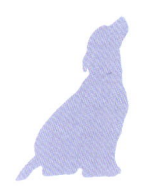

FOR DOGS

Apply the following two combinations 2–3 times daily. Alternate combinations each day. Combination 1: Apply 1 drop each Frankincense, Sandalwood, Geranium, Lavender and Myrrh in 2 tsp. carrier oil. Combination 2: Apply 1 drop each Frankincense, Cardamom, Copaiba, Pink Pepper and Lavender in 2 tsp. carrier oil. Apply 1–2 drops Digestive Blend in 1 tsp. carrier oil or a pre-diluted roll-on bottle 2–3 times daily or as needed.

Apply 1–2 drops Massage Blend in 1 tsp. carrier oil 2–3 times daily or as needed.

Ailments, Conditions, and Other Issues

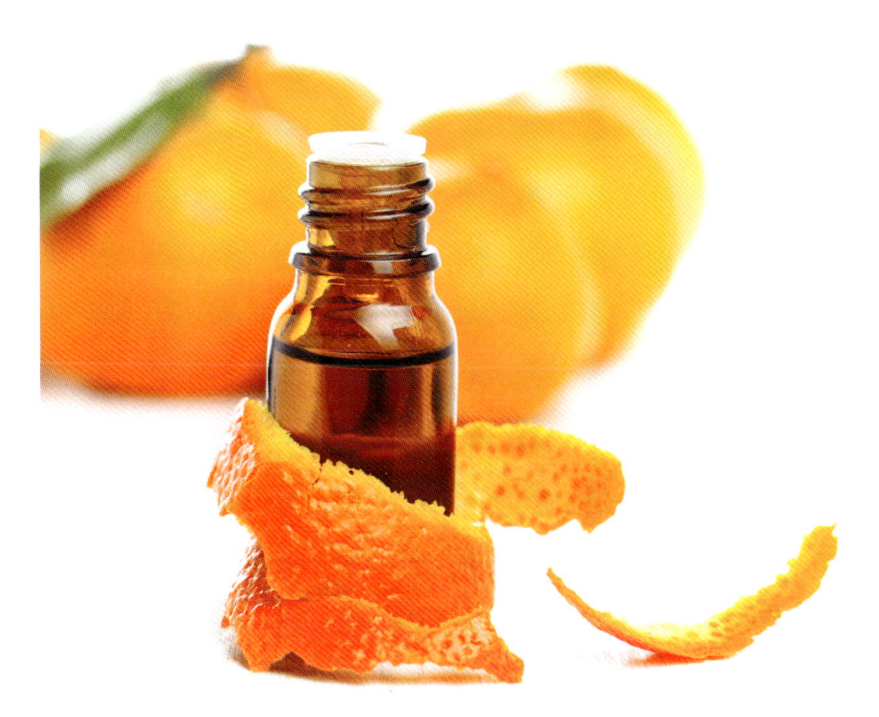

Orange

Apply 1–2 drops Grounding Blend or Restful Blend in 1 tsp. carrier oil as needed.

Administer 1 Cellular Complex (for dogs over 50 lbs.) twice daily with food. For dogs 25–50 lbs., administer 1 drop Cellular Complex 2–4 times daily with food. For smaller dogs under 25 lbs., administer 1 drop Cellular Complex twice daily with food.

Administer 1 Copaiba Softgel (for dogs over 30 lbs.) 1–2 times daily. For smaller dogs, insert a toothpick in the regulator cap of Copaiba and add this amount of oil to the food 1–2 times daily.

Insert a toothpick in the regulator cap of Grapefruit or Lemon oil and and add this amount of oil to the food 1–2 times daily.

Diffuse Protective Blend, Frankincense, and Lemon or Grapefruit, for 20–30 minutes 2–3 times daily.

Diffuse Restful Blend for 20–30 minutes 2–3 times daily.

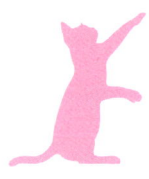

FOR CATS

Apply 1 drop each Frankincense, Sandalwood, Geranium, Lavender and Myrrh in 4 tsp. carrier oil 2–3 times daily.

Apply 1–2 drops Digestive Blend in 2 tsp. carrier oil or a pre-diluted roll-on bottle 2–3 times daily or as needed. Apply 1 drop Massage Blend in 2 tsp. carrier oil 2–3 times daily or as needed.

Apply 1–2 drops Grounding Blend or Restful Blend in 2 tsp. carrier oil as needed.

Diffuse Protective Blend, Frankincense, and Bergamot for 20–30 minutes 2–3 times daily.

Diffuse Restful Blend for 20–30 minutes 2–3 times daily.

Add Digestive Blend and/or Copaiba and Lavender to the litter box as described in Litter Box Power (See Recipes: Litter Box Power).

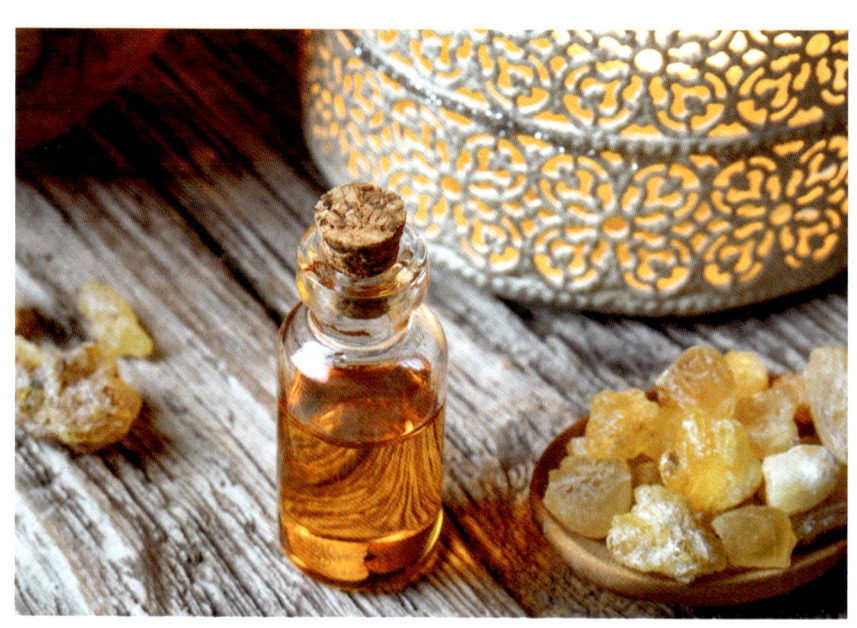

Frankincense

Ailments, Conditions, and Other Issues

CANINE COGNITIVE DISORDER

Elderly pets may develop "old dog dimentia" termed Canine Cognitive Disorder or CCD. A pet suffering from CCD may seem anxious, lost or confused,even in familiar surroundings (See Anxiety and Stress). Additional signs include inability to sleep, pacing or wandering, and staring aimlessly. Older pets often develop incontinence, loss of urine or loss of control of their bladder in which they may be unaware that they are urinating. Owners often discover puddles or wet areas where the pet has been sleeping or resting (See Urinary Conditions). Dogs afflicted with CCD affect the entire household by disrupting sleep, having accidents indoors, and frustrating their loving family.

Pets have a very sensitive sense of smell, and smell has been closely linked with memory, probably moreso than any of the other senses. A combination of essential oil blends and single oils may be helpful for CCD and triggering memory and may safely be used to complement traditional therapy without side effects or interactions. Restful Blend is perfect for inducing sleep and restfulness. Grounding blend is useful for reducing stress and anxiety. The third component of essential oil therapy for CCD is Frankincense. Frankincense is considered the "life force oil" and is helpful for many neurologic disorders. Three other single oils which are very effective are Copaiba, Bergamot and Lavender. Within a short period of time, your pet and the whole family will feel more at ease by using essential oils.

An oral supplement of Copaiba offers powerful antioxidants, neurological and immune system support and helps to relieve anxiety.

Maintaining a predictable routine, feeding a healthy diet and supplementing with higher quantities of antioxidants, Omega3 fatty acids, l-carnitine, probioticsand SAMe are all important for stability in CCD patients. The use of probiotics have been found to reduce anxiety in dogs, particularly by reducing the stress hormone cortisol.

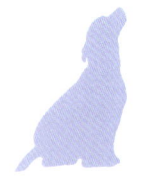

FOR DOGS

Option 1: Apply 1 drop each of Grounding Blend, Lavender and Frankincense in 1 tsp. carrier oil 2 or more times during the day. Apply 1-2 drops Restful Blend in 1 tsp. carrier oil and/or diffuse in the evening.

Option 2: Apply 1 drop each Grounding Blend, Lavender and Frankincense in 1 tsp. carrier oil 2 or more times during the day. Apply 1 drop each Copaiba and Bergamot in 1 tsp. carrier oil and/or diffuse in the evening.

Administer 1 Copaiba Softgel (for dogs over 30 lbs) 1–2 times daily. For smaller dogs, insert a toothpick in the regulator cap of Copaiba and add this amount of oil to the food 1–2 times daily. Administer 1 Restful Blend Softgel (for dogs over 15 lbs) 1–2 times daily (Restful Blend oil should not be given orally).

In addition to high quality nutrition and essential oils, several supplements have shown improvement in signs of CCD Supplement higher quantities of antioxidants, Omega-3 fatty acids, l-carnitine, probiotics and SAMe.

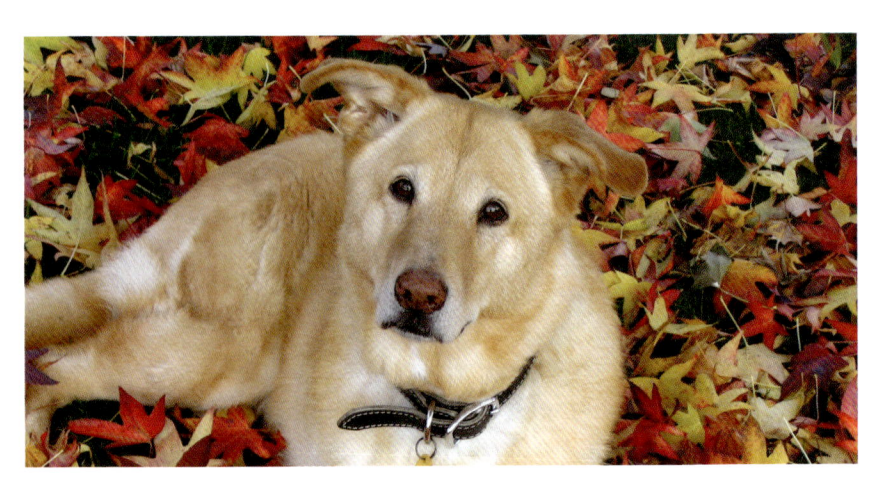

Ailments, Conditions, and Other Issues

CHEWING

Although it is normal for puppies to chew, chewing can quickly damage your furniture, your home, and your belongings and can cause harm to the puppy. Chewing is a normal part of a puppies' emotional development, and the development of their jaws and teeth. Puppies, like infants and toddlers, explore their world by putting objects into their mouths. Puppies may teethe for 6–8 months, which can create some oral discomfort. Chewing not only facilitates teething, but also helps gums feel better (See Dental Care).
As adults, chewing is relaxing, enjoyable and serves a physical need. However, adult dogs should understand what is permissible and not permissible to chew. Some dogs may not have been clearly taught what to chew and what not to chew as a puppy.

Adult dogs may engage in destructive chewing for a number of reasons. In order to deal with this behavior, you must first determine why your dog is chewing.

Possible reasons for destructive chewing include:
Boredom
Separation anxiety
Fear-related behavior
Attention-seeking behavior
Lack of proper training

Important! You may need to consult a behavior professional for help with both separation anxiety and fear-related behaviors. Most puppies and dogs benefit from training classes or the help of a private trainer or behaviorist. Discuss your concerns with your veterinarian.

Once you have determined the cause of the chewing applying and diffusing essential oils may be helpful (see Anxiety and Stress,

Separation Anxiety, Obsessive Compulsive Disorder). To deter chewing behavior, apply diluted Cassia (a hot oil), Black Pepper (a hot oil) or citrus oils to the locations and things your puppy or dog likes to chew. If chewing continues, increase the amount of essential oils applied.

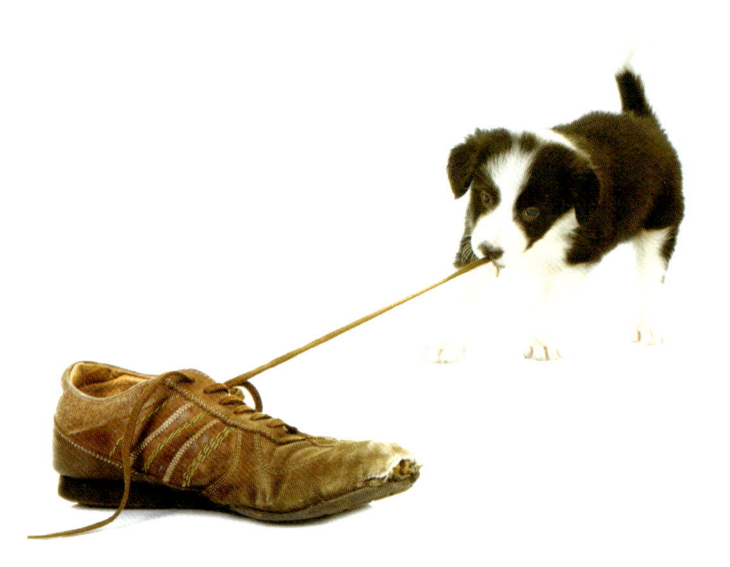

Chew Deterrent Spray with Essential Oils

Ingredients
5–6 drops of Cassia Essential Oil
or Black Pepper Essential Oil
or Citrus Essential Oil
4 oz. water
Glass or plastic spray bottle*

Instructions
Add essential oils to a 4 oz. glass or plastic spray bottle and fill with water. Shake the bottle well before use. Test the spray on a hidden area of your furniture (or other object which your puppy/dog likes to chew) to ensure it will not stain or mark the item. Spray generously and reapply as the smell wears off. If the spray does not seem to be working well, add more of the essential oil or prepare the Chew Deterrent Spray with a different hot essential oil.

CONSTIPATION

Constipation in pets is nearly always due to a poor diet. Obesity increases your pets' risk of constipation.

Feeding your pet a healthy diet, increasing fiber intake and hydration and supplementing with a probiotic can help to decrease constipation in your pet.

A high quality diet is vitally important. If the pet food is dry, consider adding warm water to the food to soften it and add moisture. Add fiber in the form of psyllium powder, fruits and vegetables (avoid grapes, raisins, garlic and onions). A daily probiotic powder or capsule will support a healthy digestive system and immune system.

Essential oils are a natural way to restore normal bowel function. The best way to apply essential oils for constipation is to massage your pet's lower abdomen with Digestive Blend daily. If the condition persists for more than one day, add Myrrh and Lavender to your daily regimen. Research has shown that stress can affect how the digestive system functions and can cause constipation. Keeping your pet calm will help him or her to feel more comfortable. Diffuse Restful Blend, Reassuring Blend or Lavender daily.

Do not give your pet any over the counter constipation medication or mineral oil. If the condition persists for more than 2–3 days, see your veterinarian. Your veterinarian may recommend a special diet and other therapies.

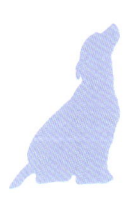

FOR DOGS

Apply 1–2 drops of Digestive Blend diluted in 1 tsp. carrier oil or a pre-diluted roll-on bottle topically up to 4 times daily. If possible, apply and massage the oil into your pet's lower abdomen for 5–7 minutes.

If the condition persists, for more than 1 day apply 1 drop each Digestive Blend, Lavender and Myrrh in 1 tsp. carrier oil up to 4 times daily and massage the oils into the lower abdomen for 5–7 minutes.

Diffuse Restful Blend, Reassuring Blend or Lavender for 20–30 minutes 2–3 times daily.

Feed your pet a high quality diet and add water and fiber to your pet's food (avoid grapes, raisins, garlic and onions). Supplement with Omega-3 and probiotics.

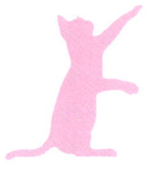

FOR CATS

Apply 1 drop Digestive Blend diluted in 2 tsp. carrier oil or a pre-diluted roll-on bottle 1–2 times daily and massage the abdomen for 5 minutes.

If the condition persists, apply 1 drop each Digestive Blend, Lavender and Myrrh in 2 tsp. carrier oil up to 4 times daily and massage the oils into the lower abdomen for 5–7 minutes.

Add Digestive Blend to the litter box as described in Litter Box Power (See Recipes: Litter Box Power).

Diffuse Restful Blend, Reassuring Blend or Lavender for 20–30 minutes 2–3 times daily.

Feed your pet a high quality diet and add water and fiber to your pet's food (avoid grapes, raisins, garlic and onions). Supplement with Omega-3 and probiotics.

COPROPHAGIA

Coprophagia is the act of dogs eating feces. It is truly disgusting, and and it is not really understood.

Dogs eat feces, usually their own, for several reasons. One common explanation is a dietary deficiency. We may think our pets are spoiled and well fed, but this may not necessarily be the case. The quality of pet food varies greatly and the pet food market is vast. When choosing a pet food, look for a food in which the first ingredient is protein and in which all of the ingredients are recognizable as food rather then a list of chemicals and fillers. Often, a puppy who has had an accident is trying to avoid getting caught. The last explanation is that this awful behavior has become a habit for the dog. A habit can develop from boredom, lack of stimulation and activity, or stress and anxiety (See Anxiety and Stress).

> *"There is no psychiatrist in the world like a puppy licking your face."*
>
> *- Ben Williams*

First, be sure to feed a high quality diet and supplement with Omega-3 and probiotics. Further support good digestion with Digestive Blend applied twice daily. Diffuse calming essential oils such as Restful Blend, Grounding Blend, Comforting Blend or Reassuring Blend to reduce stress and anxiety.

Ensure your dog is getting adequate exercise, mental stimulation and attention. Discuss this condition with your veterinarian and trainer.

SpOil Your Pet

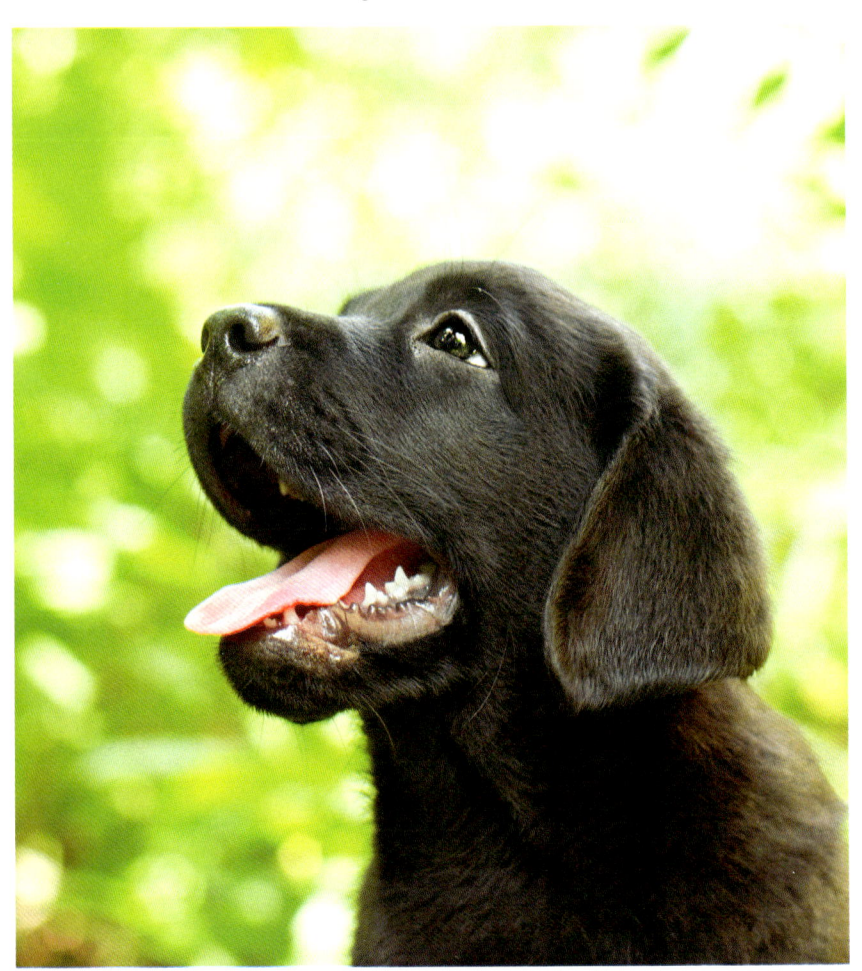

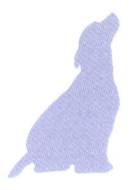

FOR DOGS

Apply 1–2 drops of Digestive Blend diluted in 1 tsp. carrier oil or a pre-diluted roll-on bottle twice daily.

Apply 1 drop of either Restful Blend, Grounding Blend, Comforting Blend or Reassuring Blend diluted in 1 tsp. carrier oil or diffuse for 20–30 minutes 2–3 times daily.

Feed a healthy diet and supplement with Omega- 3 and probiotics.

CUSHING'S DISEASE (HYPERADRENOCORTICISM)

Cushing's disease is characterized by an overproduction of cortisol which is commonly known as the stress hormone. Cortisol is produced by the adrenal glands under the control of the "master gland", the pituitary gland and are located near the kidneys. Cotisol is an important hormone and helps the body to cope in times of stress, regulates body weight, blood sugar and skin health (See Anxiety and Stress, Nutrition). Too much cortisol can weaken the immune system, leading to other diseases and infections.

This disease is often seen in older dogs and rarely in cats. Signs of Cushing's disease include increased thirst and urination, an insatiable appetite, a pot-bellied appearance, dry, thin, fragile skin, increased pigmentation of the skin, excessive panting, restlessness and recurrent skin or bladder infections. If you observe any of these signs, consult your veterinarian for a thorough physical exam and diagnostic testing such as blood work, ultrasound and urinalysis. The disease is confirmed with a secondary blood test.

Approximately 85% of cases of Cushing's disease are the result of a tumor on the pituitary gland, located at the base of the brain and 15% are due to a tumor on the adrenal gland. Abdominal ultrasound can help to locate an adrenal tumor. These tumors may be benign or malignant.

Another cause of Cushing's disease is due to excessive or prolonged use of steroid medication. Steroid are commonly prescribed for auto-immune disease, allergies, seizures, cancers, and inflammatory conditions. This class of hyperadrenocorticism is called iatrogenic. In many cases, the use of essential oils can replace steroid medication.

Depending on the type of Cushing's disease which develops, your pet may live several years with attentive veterinary care. Cushing's disease either originating from the pituitary or adrenal gland, is managed by using a traditional medication or, more naturally with Melatonin and Flax Seed supplements. In some cases of adrenal tumors, surgery may be chosen to remove the tumor. In cases of Cushing's which is due to steroid medication, discontinuation of the medication may alleviate the symptoms of Cushing's. However, this should only be done under the guidance of your veterinarian to safely monitor steroid withdrawal and to prevent your pet from having the symptoms of the original disease for which the steroids were prescribed.

Essential oils can help to support your pet's pituitary and adrenal glands and balance hormones. Some oils to consider include Detoxification Blend, Geranium, Fennel, Ylang Ylang, Frankincense, Copaiba, and Black Pepper. We suggest applying a combination of Detoxification Blend, Geranium, Frankincense, Black Pepper and Copaiba. Diffuse Ylang Ylang, Invigorating Blend and Restful Blend for a feeling of calm and balance. To support the immune system and maintain overall health, diffuse Protective Blend. Continue to support overall health by feeding a high quality diet and supplementing with Omega-3 and probiotics. The use of probiotics have been found to reduce anxiety in dogs, particularly by reducing the stress hormone cortisol.

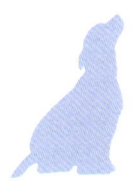

FOR DOGS

Apply 1 drop each Detoxification Blend, Geranium, Frankincense, Black Pepper and Copaiba in 2 tsp. carrier oil twice daily.

Diffuse two of the following Ylang Ylang, Invigorating Blend and Restful Blend for 20–30 minutes 2–3 times daily.

Diffuse Protective Blend for 20–30 minutes 2–3 times daily.

Feed your dog a high quality diet supplemented with Omega-3 and probiotics.

CUTS AND SCRAPES

Active, curious pets often get into trouble or have small accidents. Minor cuts can happen very easily. Examples include cutting toe pads, slipping on the ice, stepping on rocks outside, and broken toenails. Contact your veterinarian if the cut is actively bleeding, will not stop bleeding, is deeper than the surface of the skin or if your pet is limping due to the injury, or continues to lick at a wound for more than 1–2 days. We do not advise bandaging wounds without the recommendation of your veterinarian.

The basic steps for treating a minor cut or scrape are:

* Stop the bleeding. Apply pressure if necessary.
* Clean the wound. Remove any foreign material. (If the wound is deep, contact your veterinarian.)
* Apply an antibiotic essential oil.
* Keep the wound clean and dry.
* Monitor for signs of infection such as a yellow or green discharge or odor.

Essential oils are ideal choices for any of these steps because they have cleansing, antibacterial and pain relieving properties. In addition, they are calming for both you and your pet in a stressful situation.

- In the event of a minor, superficial wound, first stop the bleeding. Many times, applying pressure for a few minutes is effective. If additional help is needed, apply Helichrysum to aid in blood clotting. Do not use Helichrysum if there is a puncture wound.

- After the bleeding has stopped, immediately clean the wound with Gentle Cleanser or hydrogen peroxide using gauze or cotton balls immediately. Hydrogen peroxide is an effective cleanser initially, but it is best to use it only once. Repeated use of hydrogen peroxide can delay healing. Continue cleaning the wound with Gentle Cleanser 1–2 times daily.

- Apply 1–2 drops Lavender essential oil in carrier oil. Lavender is a natural antiseptic and pain reliever. Simultaneously, the aroma of Lavender is calming. After applying Lavender directly to the wound, rub 2–3 drops in the palms of your hands, and let your pet inhale the soothing fragrance.

- Several other essential oils that have antibacterial properties including Frankincense, Myrrh, and Geranium can be used. Add 1 drop each Lavender, Frankincense, Myrrh, and Geranium to a bowl of warm water, and apply a compress to the affected area twice daily. Apply 1 drop each Lavender, Frankincense, Myrrh and Geranium diluted in carrier oil to the wound to prevent infection. Repeat the application of the antibacterial essential oil combination every 4–6 hours for the first 3 days. After 3 days, continue to apply the antibacterial essential oils 1–2 times daily. Consult your veterinarian if the wound does not appear to be healing, has a persistent discharge, develops an odor or is painful.

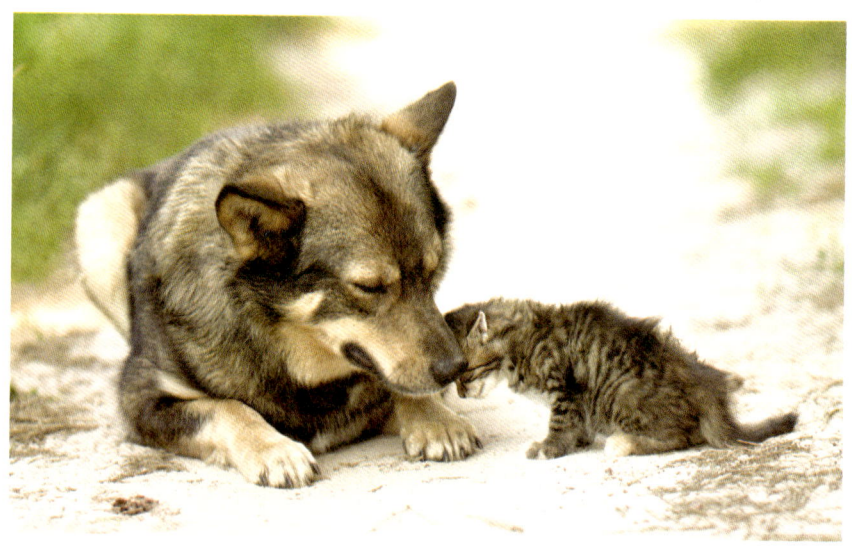

- Beginning on day 4, apply Helichrysum combined with the antibacterial oils daily during the healing process to reduce or eliminate scarring.

- Keep the wound clean and dry, and protect it by restricting your pet's time outdoors.

Ailments, Conditions, and Other Issues

- Continue to diffuse Restful Blend or Lavender alternating with Protective Blend to help calm the household and reduce the risk of infection for several days. Add Lavender to the litter box as described in Litter Box Power (See Recipes: Litter Box Power).
- Continue high quality nutrition and supplement with Omega -3 and Probiotics.

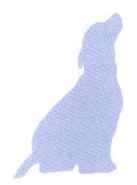

FOR DOGS

Stop the bleeding with pressure for 3–5 minutes. If bleeding does not subside, apply 1 drop Helichrysum in 1 tsp. carrier oil. **If bleeding persists, call your veterinarian.**

Clean the wound with Gentle Cleanser or Hydrogen peroxide initially. Clean with Gentle Cleanser daily during the healing process.

Apply 1 drop each Lavender, Frankincense, Myrrh and Geranium in 2 tsp carrier oil every 4–6 hours for the first 3 days.

After 3 days, continue to apply the antibacterial essential oils twice daily.

Beginning on day 4, add 1 drop Helichrysum to the antibacterial oil combination and apply twice daily.

Diffuse Restful Blend or Lavender for 20–30 minutes twice daily.

Diffuse Protective Blend 20–30 minutes twice daily.

Continue high quality nutrition and supplements with Omega-3 and probiotics.

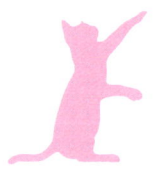

FOR CATS

Stop the bleeding with pressure for 3–5 minutes. If bleeding does not subside, apply 1 drop Helichrysum in 2 tsp. carrier oil. **If bleeding persists, call your veterinarian.**

Clean the wound with Gentle Cleanser or Hydrogen peroxide initially. Clean with Gentle Cleanser daily during the healing process.

Apply 1 drop each Lavender, Frankincense Myrrh, and Geranium in 4 tsp. carrier oil repeat every 4–6 hours for the first 3 days.

After 3 days, continue to apply the antibacterial essential oils 2 times daily.

Beginning on day 4, add 1 drop Helichrysum to the antibacterial oil combination and apply twice daily.

Diffuse Restful Blend or Lavender for 20–30 minutes twice daily.

Diffuse Protective Blend 20–30 minutes twice daily.

Add Lavender to the litter box as described in Litter Box Power (See Recipes: Litter Box Power).

Continue high quality nutrition and supplement with Omega -3 and Probiotics.

Gentle Cleanser

Ingredients
4 oz. Castile soap or unscented natural foaming soap
2 drops Roman Chamomile Essential Oil
2 drops Lavender Essential Oil
Glass or Plastic Container*

Instructions
Add essential oils to glass or plastic container. Top with soap. Shake the bottle well before use. Lather and rinse well.

Ailments, Conditions, and Other Issues

DEMODEX/MANGE

Demodectic Mange, referred to as Demodex, is a mite infestation commonly seen in puppies, young adult dogs and old dogs. Demodectic mites live in the hair follicles and are not contagious to people. Demodex is often associated with a suppressed immune system.

Signs of demodex include patches of hair loss, redness of the skin and crusty eruptions of the skin. Some dogs are itchy with this condition. Your veterinarian will diagnose demodex with a physical exam and microscopic examination of skin scrapings. Demodex may be treated with oral or topical medication and medicated shampoo. Complete cure may take weeks to months.

Essential oils complement traditional therapy. Apply Lavender, Geranium, Cleansing Blend and Helichrysum daily to the affected areas or by petting. Apply Healing Salve daily. Bathe weekly to twice weekly with Antiseptic Shampoo with 3 drops Cleansing Blend added. Feed your pet a high quality diet and supplement with Omega-3 and probiotics.

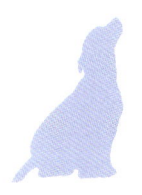

FOR DOGS

Apply 1 drop each of Cleansing Blend, Geranium, Lavender, and Helichrysum in 2 tsp. carrier oil to affected areas or by petting twice daily.

Apply Healing Salve 1–2 times twice daily to localized lesions.

Bathe with Antiseptic Shampoo with added Cleansing Blend 1–2 times weekly.

Feed a high quality diet and supplement with Omega-3 and probiotics.

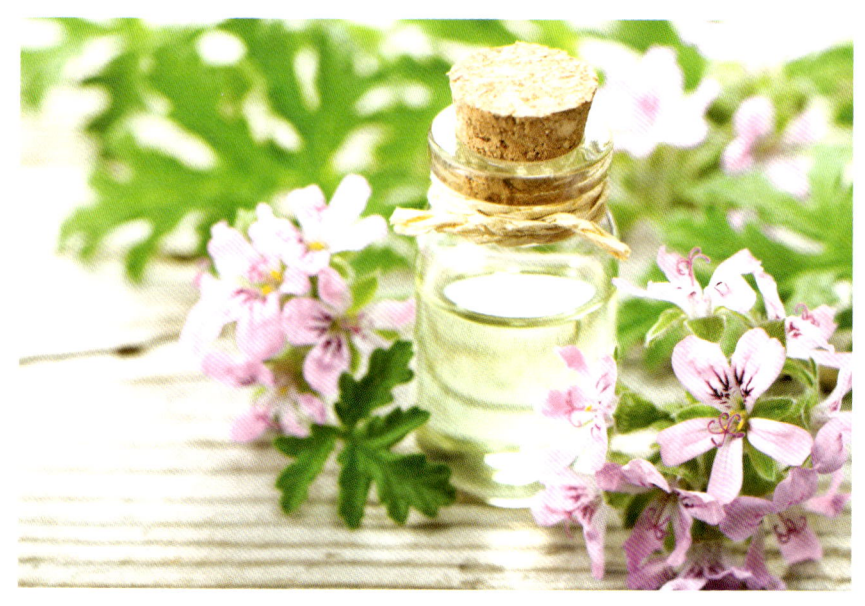

Geranium

Antiseptic Shampoo

Ingredients
110 oz. Water
2 oz. Aloe Vera
1 Tbsp. Castile soap
2 drops Myrrh Essential Oil
2 drops Lavender Essential Oil
2 drops Geranium Essential Oil
2 drops Cleansing Essential Oil Blend
Glass or Plastic Bottle
Instructions
Add essential oils to an empty bottle. Add castile soap, aloe vera juice and water. Shake the bottle well before use. Lather and rinse well.

Healing Salve

Ingredients

8 oz. Cold-Pressed Organic Coconut Oil
1 oz. Beeswax
2 drops Vitamin E (optional)
10 drops Lavender Essential Oil
5 drops Myrrh Essential Oil
3 drops Helichrysum Essential Oil
Glass Jars, Tin Containers or Plastic Bottle*

Instructions

Place the coconut oil and beeswax over a double –boiler, and gently warm over low heat until the beeswax melts. Remove from heat and add the essential oils and Vitamin E oil, (if using). Quickly pour the mixture into glass jars, tins, or plastic containers and allow to cool completely. Store salve in a cool location where it will not re-melt and re-solidify. When stored correctly, salve will last for 1–3 years. Yields 8 oz.

"Money can buy you a fine dog, but only love can make him wag his tail."

- Kinky Friedman

DENTAL CARE

Dental disease affects the entire body. Caring for your pet's teeth and gums improves the quality of their life and extends it. Bacteria that accumulate in the mouth enter the bloodstream and can adversely affect the kidneys, heart and liver. Dental disease also causes terrible oral pain, bad breath and possible difficulty eating or chewing properly. Once a pet's teeth and gums are severely infected, receded or diseased (periodontal disease), extractions will most likely be needed.

In addition to oral examinations with each veterinary visit, dogs and cats should have annual dental cleanings much like our own in order to maintain healthy teeth and gums. Performing routine veterinary examinations, regular dental cleanings and good home care will prevent the progression of periodontal disease.

> *"Dogs are not our whole life, but they make our lives whole."*
>
> *- Roger Caras*

Home care is very important. It is ideal to brush your pet's teeth daily with fluoride-free toothpaste. Fluoride has been shown to have ill effects for pets. Toothpaste with essential oils is very easy to make at home using a combination of baking soda, bentonite clay, coconut oil and any of the following essential oils- Myrrh, Protective Blend or Peppermint (See Homemade Doggie Toothpaste recipe below). Commercial toothpastes made for pets are available in flavors such as beef, poultry, peanut butter and fish. When choosing a toothpaste for your pet be sure to use a product that does not contain Xylitol, as it is toxic to dogs and cats. Brushing may be difficult for some dogs and for most cats to accept. So, the next best option is to offer safe and effective dental chews daily. Avoid giving your dog real bones as they can fracture teeth, splinter or become lodged in their mouth or throat. A third option is to add a veterinary recommended dental water additive in the drinking water to delay tartar accumulation. Any of these three methods of home dental care may be combined.

Don't be discouraged that tartar still builds up on your pet's teeth. There is nothing that will prevent tartar 100%. Even with the best of home care, your pet will still benefit from dental cleanings on an annual basis. Feed a high quality diet and supplement with Omega-3 and probiotics.

Essential oils can help maintain a strong immune system, fight bacteria and reduce pain.

For dogs and cats, apply Myrrh, Copaiba and Helichrysum once to twice daily. For dogs with more advanced dental disease, administer an oral preparation of Copaiba to support the immune system and decrease inflammation. Diffuse Protective Blend and Lemon, alternating oils every few days.

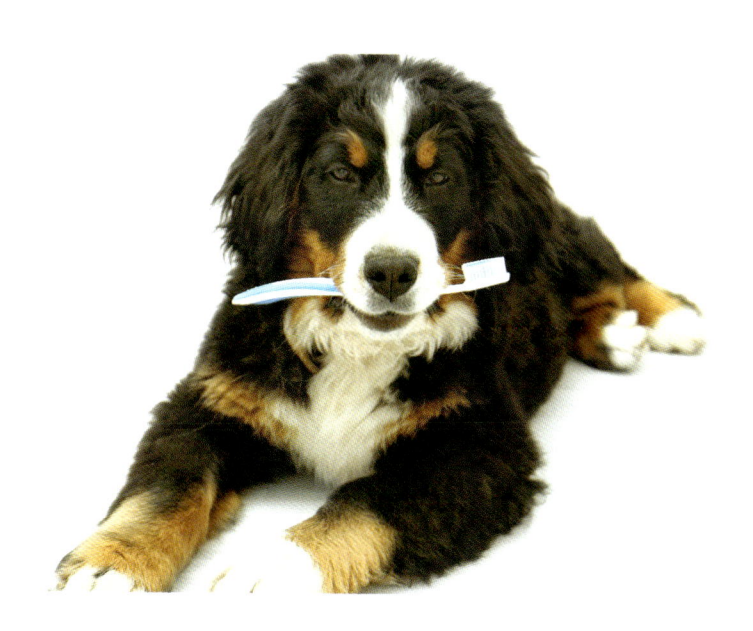

SpOil Your Pet

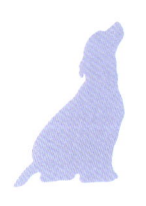

FOR DOGS

Apply 1 drop each Myrrh, Copaiba and Helichrysum in 1 tsp. carrier oil 1–2 times daily.

Administer 1 Copaiba Softgel (for dogs over 30 lbs.) 1–2 times daily. For smaller dogs, insert a toothpick in the regulator cap of Copaiba and add this amount of oil to the food 1–2 times daily.

Diffuse Protective Blend or Lemon for 20–30 minutes 2–3 times daily, alternating oils every few days.

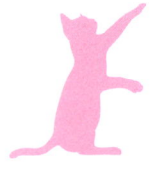

FOR CATS

Apply 1 drop each Myrrh, Copaiba, and Helichrysum in 2 tsp. carrier oil 1–2 times daily.

Diffuse Protective Blend or Lemon for 20–30 minutes 2–3 times daily, alternating oils every few days.

Homemade Doggie Toothpaste

Ingredients
1 Tbsp. Baking Soda
1 Tbsp. Bentonite Clay
1 Tbsp. Solid Organic Coconut Oil
1 drop Peppermint Essential Oil
1 drop Myrrh Essential Oil
Glass or Plastic Container*

Instructions
Add the coconut oil to a glass bowl and whisk well. Add the baking soda and bentonite clay to the coconut oil and mix thoroughly. Add essential oils to this mixture. Store in a glass or plastic container in a cool place. Makes a 1 month supply if used daily.

Ailments, Conditions, and Other Issues

DIABETES

Diabetes mellitus is a disease in which blood sugar levels are abnormally high. Diabetes is characterized by a lack of production of insulin from the pancreas or the body's resistance or inability to use insulin. Insulin is a hormone that regulates blood sugar levels. When blood sugar levels rise, such as after a meal, the pancreas secretes insulin to reduce the blood sugar and enable the cells to utilize the sugar for energy. In pets with Diabetes, blood sugar levels remain high affecting overall metabolism and health.

Causes of diabetes in dogs include heredity, infection, obesity, and pancreatitis. In cats, potential causes of diabetes include obesity and protein accumulation in the cells of the pancreas. (See Obesity, Organ Support)

Common signs of diabetes are excessive thirst, excessive urination, increased appetite, and weight loss (See Urinary Conditions). Diabetic pets are also susceptible to increased infections and may have difficulty healing. (See Cuts and Scrapes)

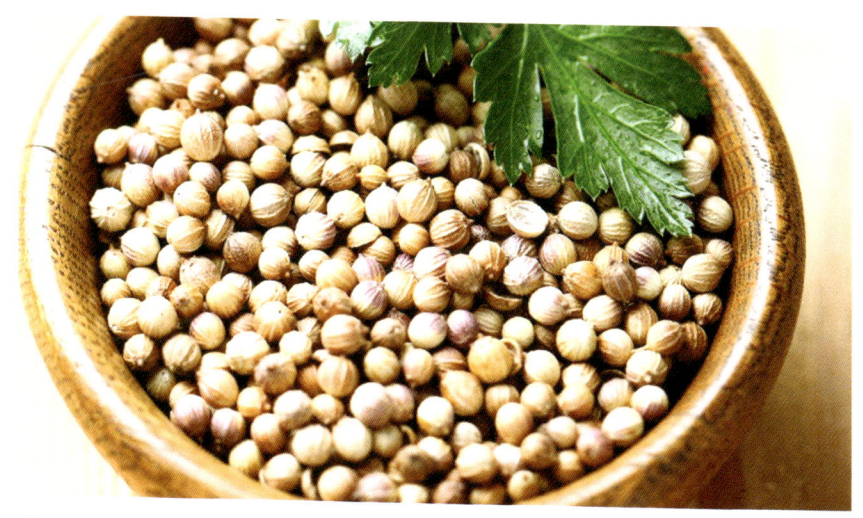

Coriander

In addition to insulin therapy guided by your veterinarian, several essential oils are helpful to regulate blood sugar, improve metabolism, slow the absorption of carbohydrates and heal secondary infections The use of essential oils in diabetes may reduce or eliminate the amount of insulin needed.

Apply a combination of Coriander, Myrrh, and Geranium. Copaiba, and Ylang Ylang may be used for additional support. Monitor your pet and work closely with your veterinarian to ensure proper blood glucose/sugar levels are maintained. Apply or diffuse Grounding Blend or Restful Blend twice daily to reduce anxiety and stress. Diffuse Protective Blend twice daily to support the immune system. For cats. add Myrrh or Copaiba and Ylang Ylang to the litter box (See Recipes: Litter Box Power).

For many diabetic pets, a change in diet, exercise and subsequent weight loss may reduce and/or eliminate the need for insulin and improve your pet's health overall. Continue to supplement with Omega-3 and probiotics.

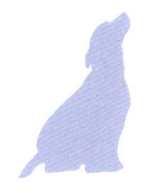

FOR DOGS

Apply 1 drop each Coriander, Myrrh, and Geranium in 1 tsp. carrier oil 2–3 times daily.

Apply 1 drop Grounding Blend or Restful Blend in 1 tsp carrier oil twice daily.

Diffuse Grounding Blend or Restful Blend for 20–30 minutes 2–3 times daily.

Diffuse Protective Blend for 20–30 minutes 2–3 times daily.

Feed a high quality diet and continue to supplement with Omega-3 and probiotics.

Ailments, Conditions, and Other Issues

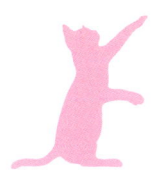

FOR CATS

Apply 1 drop each Coriander, Myrrh, and Geranium in 2 tsp. carrier oil and apply twice daily.

Apply 1 drop Grounding Blend or Restful Blend in 2 tsp. carrier oil twice daily.

Diffuse Grounding Blend or Restful Blend for 20–30 minutes 2–3 times daily.

Diffuse Protective Blend for 20–30 minutes 2–3 times daily.

Feed a high quality diet and continue to supplement with Omega-3 and probiotics.

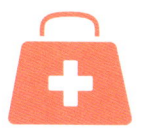

IT IS IMPORTANT TO MAINTAIN CLOSE CONTACT WITH YOUR VETERINARIAN IF YOU ARE USING ESSENTIAL OILS TO SUPPORT YOUR DIABETIC PET.

DIARRHEA AND VOMITING

Diarrhea and vomiting may have a number of causes. Very commonly, dogs and cats encounter short-lived viruses, stomach bugs or intestinal parasites (See Intestinal Parasites). Dogs may chew on leaves or grass outside, resulting in mild diarrhea, gas and an upset stomach. Occasionally, pets misbehave by getting into the garbage. Table food may also upset the digestive system.

Often, pets do not tolerate abrupt changes in diet. When changing your pet's brand of food, flavor or formula, introduce the new food gradually over 5–7 days to ease the transition and avoid diarrhea and vomiting.

Stress also can cause stomach upset. What causes feelings of stress in our pets? New situations, moving, large gatherings, guests in the home, a new baby, changes in work schedules, traveling, and loss of an owner or a companion are all examples of stressful instances (See Stress and Anxiety, Grief and Loss).Under these circumstances, Digestive Blend and Myrrh are quite helpful.

For Dogs, apply Digestive Blend and Myrrh topically to your dog several times daily to reduce symptoms. Rub the oil on your pet's belly or anywhere on the body. It will be absorbed and work even if it is applied to the back. Diffuse Protective Blend to support the immune system. Diffuse Restful Blend or Reassuring Blend to maintain emotional balance.

For cats, place Digestive blend and Myrrh oil in the palm of your hands and rub your hands together to allow most of the oil to absorb. Apply by petting your cat daily or as needed. Rub the oil on your pet's belly or anywhere on the body, and it will be absorbed and work even if it is applied to the back. Diffuse Protective Blend to support the immune system. Diffuse Restful Blend or Reassuring Blend to maintain emotional balance.

For both dogs and cats, withhold food initially for 12–24 hours, then offer a bland diet of boiled chicken, low fat chopped meat, rice, cottage cheese or yogurt. Continue the bland diet in smaller, more frequent meals until signs of diarrhea or vomiting have passed for at least three days. Then, gradually convert back to your pet's healthy, regular diet. Once vomiting has ceased, continue to administer your pet's probiotic. If your pet refuses the bland diet or vomits everything he or she eats or drinks, contact your veterinarian.

In all cases of diarrhea and vomiting, your pet is losing important fluids. It is very important to maintain proper hydration to allow all the organs of the body to function well. Offer your pet water and add additional water to the homemade rice. If your pet is not eating and drinking well or has suffered several days of vomiting or diarrhea, dehydration may develop and he or she may need to be treated by your veterinarian.

A word of caution: If diarrhea or vomiting persists for more than 1–2 days, increases in frequency or is bloody, call your veterinarian. Severe lethargy and lack of appetite are also indications that you should contact your veterinarian. If there is any possibility that your pet may have eaten an indigestible object such as a toy, clothing, or string, seek veterinary care immediately. Several days of illness may be due to a more severe condition such as intestinal parasites, kidney or liver disease, or other metabolic disease (See Organ Support).

"What greater gift than the love of a cat."
- Charles Dickens

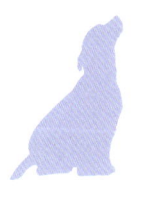

FOR DOGS

Apply 1 drop each Digestive Blend and Myrrh in 1 tsp. carrier oil 2–3 times daily as needed.

Diffuse Protective Blend for 20–30 minutes 2–3 times daily.

Diffuse Restful Blend or Reassuring Blend for 20–30 minutes 2–3 times daily.

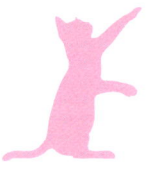

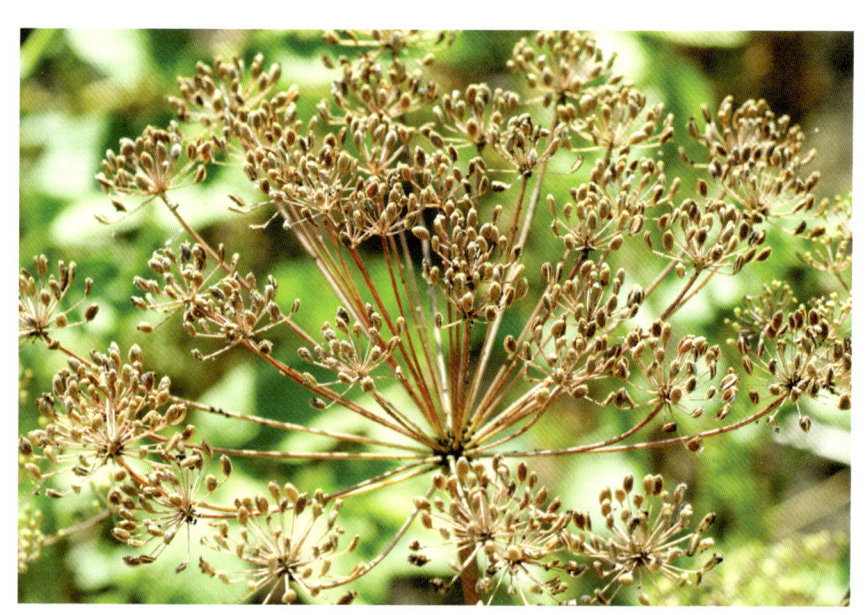

FOR CATS

Apply 1 drop each Digestive Blend and 1 drop Myrrh in 2 tsp. carrier oil 1–2 times daily.

Diffuse Protective Blend for 20–30 minutes 2–3 times daily.

Diffuse Restful Blend or Reassuring Blend for 20–30 minutes 2–3 times daily.

Fennel, found in a digestive blend

Ailments, Conditions, and Other Issues

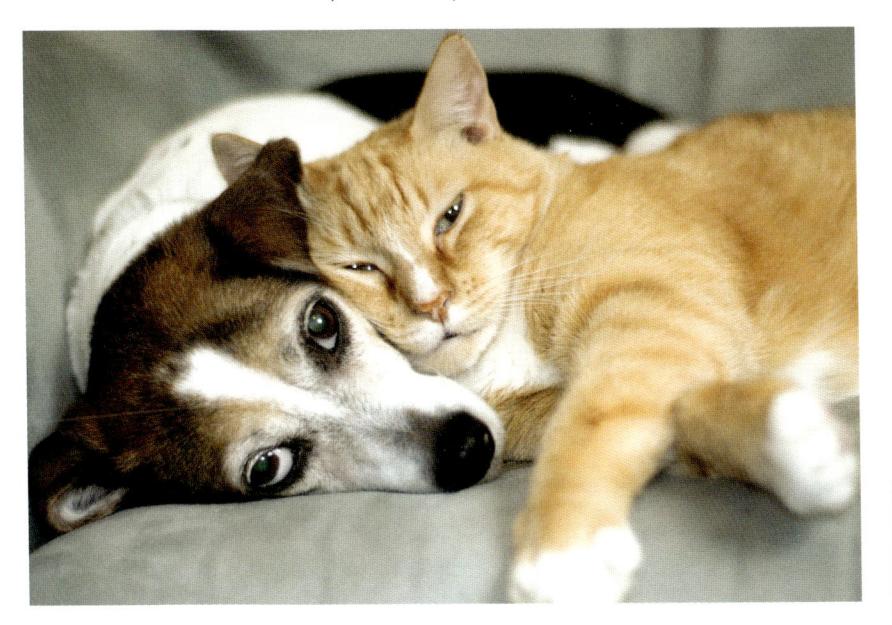

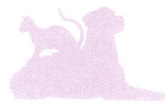

FOR DOGS & CATS

Withhold food initially for 12–24 hours, then offer a bland diet of boiled chicken, low fat chopped meat, rice, cottage cheese or yogurt. Continue the bland diet in smaller, more frequent meals until signs of diarrhea or vomiting have passed for at least three days. Then, gradually convert back to your pet's healthy, regular diet.

Once vomiting has ceased, continue to administer a probiotic.

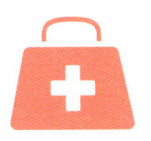

A Word of Caution: If diarrhea or vomiting persists for more than 1–2 days, increases in frequency or is bloody, call your veterinarian. If your pet refuses to eat or vomits everything he or she eats or drinks, contact your veterinarian. Severe lethargy and lack of appetite are also indications to contact your veterinarian.

DRY SKIN (SEBORRHEA SICCA)

Skin stays moist due to the production of sebum (oil). Dry skin does not naturally produce enough sebum. Pets commonly develop dry, flaky skin in the winter months from forced air heating, in the summer months from air conditioning, from poor nutrition or from over bathing. Fortunately, there are a number of essential oils that help to stimulate the production of sebum, and also balance secretions within the skin, thus helping dry skin.

Essential Oils are both calming and gentle, and help to soothe dry, itchy, and inflamed skin. Bathe your dog 1–2 times weekly with a natural shampoo adding Lavender, Roman Chamomile, and Myrrh essential oils to help soothe, calm, and repair the skin (See Recipe for Soothing Skin Shampoo below). Apply Lavender, Sandalwood, and Roman Chamomile daily. Be sure to feed your dog a high quality diet and supplement with Omega-3 and a probiotic. Cats generally do not tolerate bathing. For cats who have dry skin, we suggest applying Lavender, Sandalwood, and Roman Chamomile daily. Be sure to feed your cat a high quality diet and supplement with Omega-3 and a probiotic.

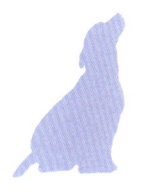

FOR DOGS

Bathe 1–2 times weekly using Soothing Skin Shampoo. Caution: When bathing with essential oils, be careful to avoid the eyes.

Dilute 1–2 drops each Lavender, Sandalwood and Roman Chamomile in 1 tsp. carrier oil and apply 1–2 times daily.

Feed a high quality diet and supplement with Omega-3 and probiotics.

Ailments, Conditions, and Other Issues

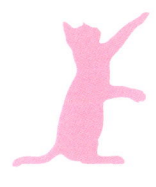

FOR CATS

We recommend you find a groomer that specializes in cats and have your groomer use the Soothing Skin Shampoo.

Dilute 1 drop eachLavender, Sandalwood and Roman Chamomile in 2 tsp. carrier oil and apply 1–2 times daily.

Feed a high quality diet and supplement with Omega-3 and probiotics.

Soothing Skin Shampoo

Ingredients
3 oz. Castile soap (available at many health and bulk food stores)
2 oz. Organic unpasteurized, unfiltered Apple Cider Vinegar
1 oz. Vegetable Glycerin
2 oz. Distilled water
3 drops Lavender Essential Oil
3 drops Roman Chamomile Essential Oil
3 drops Myrrh Essential Oil
Optional: *add 1 tsp. ground oatmeal*
*Glass or Plastic Bottle**

Instructions
Add essential oils to an empty glass or plastic bottle. Add ground oatmeal (if using). Add the apple cider vinegar, vegetable glycerin, and water to the bottle containing essential oils and oatmeal. Add the castile soap. Shake the bottle well before use.

EAR CLEANING

The first step in becoming comfortable in cleaning our pets' ears is to understand their anatomy. A dog or cat's ear canal is a long, "L" shaped tube in which the ear drum (tympanic membrane) is protected by being a distance from the surface. The ear canal has a vertical section, a nearly 90 degree turn, and a horizontal section prior to reaching the ear drum. It is quite different from our ear canal which is short and straight, and easy to touch. Because your pet's ear drum is literally inches away and past a curve, it is protected.

However, the shape of the ear canal makes dogs and cats predisposed to ear infections. The ear canal is naturally deep and dark, so any moisture (humidity, bathing, swimming, etc.) can easily contribute to an infection. The goal of cleaning your pet's ears is to maintain a dry environment that discourages the growth of bacteria and yeast. The process of cleaning your pet's ears to maintain a healthy ear canal or when they are infected is the same. The only difference is in the frequency of cleaning the ears.

Generously apply 1–3 tsp. of a safe natural ear cleaner as directed by your veterinarian and massage the ear canal (See Natural Ear Cleaner recipe below). Either pour the cleaner into the ear canal and massage, or saturate a cotton ball, place it at the top of the ear canal, and massage the ear to release the fluid. Remove the cotton ball. Proceed with wiping out the ear canal with dry cotton balls. (The cotton ball method is useful for cats.)

You will know that sufficient cleaner has been applied when a swishing sound can be heard as you massage the ear canal, loosening debris and driving it to the surface. Using cotton balls, wipe the ear canal by inserting your finger as deeply as you can. Although this sounds aggressive, your finger cannot reach the ear drum. Continue to flush the ear with cleaning solution and wipe

Ailments, Conditions, and Other Issues

with cotton balls until the canal is clean and the cotton balls are removed with very little or no debris.

After having an ear cleaning, pets will often rub their heads on the floor, rub against the furniture and shake their heads excessively. Do not worry that you have done any harm. The ears simply feel wet and different to your pet.

Note: To clean your pet's ears, you may need the support of a second person, especially for cats. Confine your pet to a small room, and make the experience as positive as possible. Treats as enticement and reward are helpful.

For cats, you may only get to wipe 2 or 3 times. That's OK. It is better to keep the atmosphere positive for a short cleaning than to struggle for quite some time.

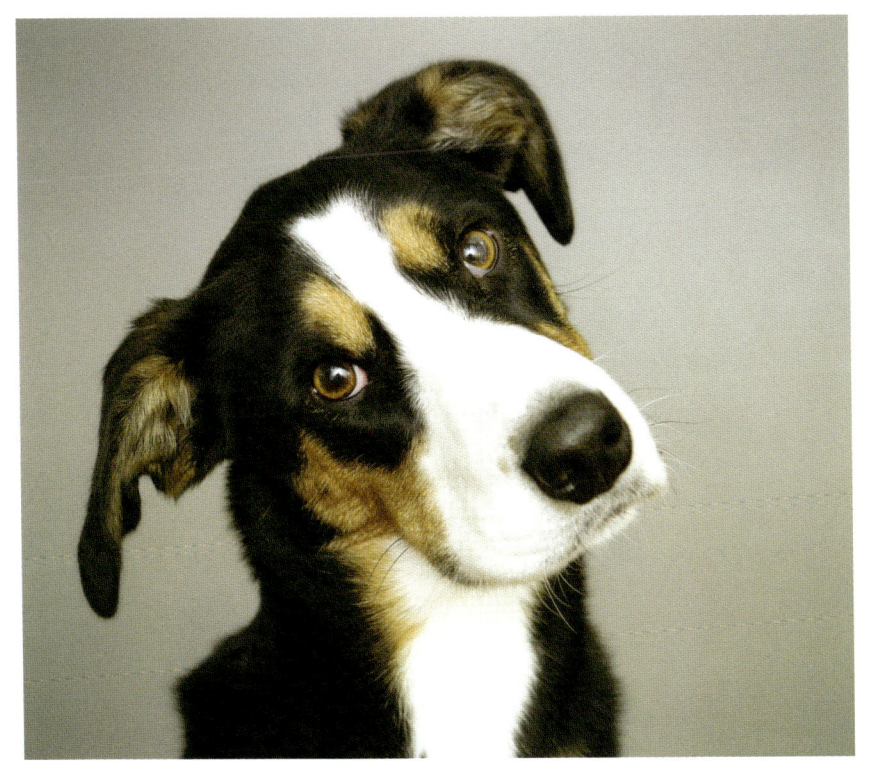

We generally recommend cleaning weekly to every two weeks based on seasonal humidity and contact with water. During an infection, the frequency of cleaning is often increased to three times weekly. Apply Lavender essential oil around the base of the ear to help calm your pet and prevent infection.

Signs of an ear infection include scratching at the ear(s), shaking his or her head, holding the head to one side, redness, inflammation, debris in the ears and an unpleasant odor from the ear(s). If your pet demonstrates severe signs of discomfort or if signs of an infection persist, contact your veterinarian.

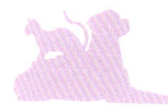

FOR DOGS & CATS

Clean ears with Natural Ear Cleaner every 1–2 weeks for maintenance or up to three times weekly for treatment of an infection.

Apply 1 drop Lavender in 1 tsp. carrier oil for dogs and 2 tsp. carrier oil in cats around the base of the ears. Do not apply essential oils directly in the ear canal.

Ailments, Conditions, and Other Issues

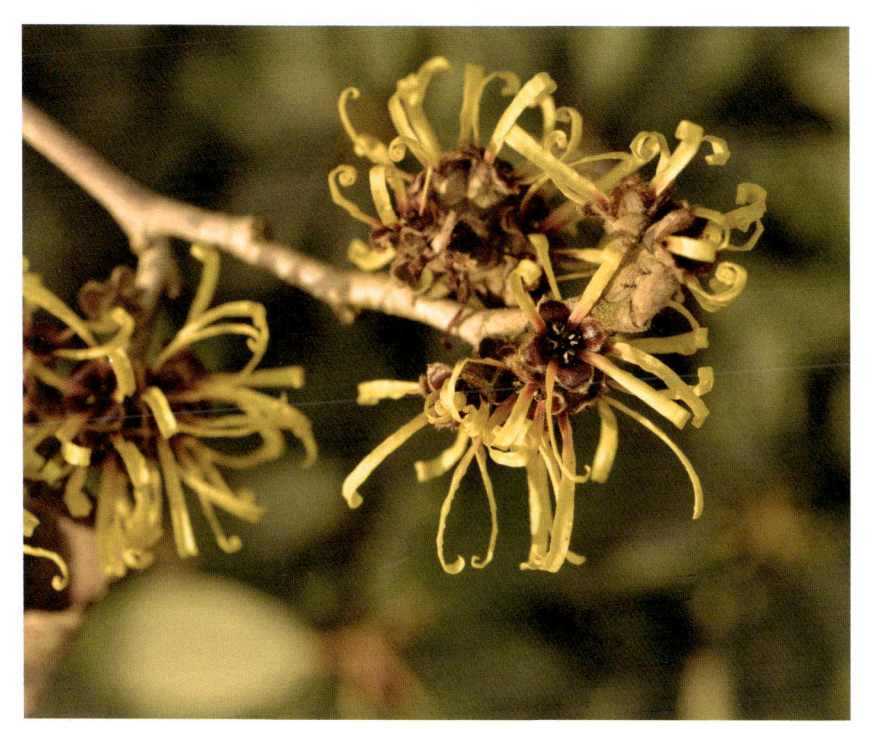

Witch Hazel

Natural Ear Cleaner

Ingredients
1 oz. Witch Hazel
1 oz. Apple Cider Vinegar

Sometimes referred to as nature's antibiotic, witch hazel can be effective in cleaning your pet's ears while protecting them from further infection. This natural remedy, produced from the leaves and bark of the North American witch hazel shrub, encourages quicker healing of minor breaks in skin and has proven anti-inflammatory properties.

Used for decades in folk medicine, apple cider vinegar has been proven to kill germs and heal naturally.

EAR INFECTIONS

Dogs and cats are particularly susceptible to ear infections due to their long, deep and curved ear canals. The dark environment coupled with moisture, due to bathing, swimming, humidity, rain, etc. provide the perfect environment for yeast and bacteria to grow. Ear infections may be prevented by properly cleaning your pet's ears regularly and especially after contact with water (See Ear Cleaning). A dog or cat may be more likely to develop ear infections as a result of allergies (seasonal, food or contact), some medical conditions, and as members of certain breeds (see Allergies). Addressing any underlying causes and feeding a high quality diet is crucial for maintaining overall health. We recommend you have your pet tested for environmental and food allergies.

> *" As every cat owner knows, nobody owns a cat."*
>
> *- Ellen Perry Berkeley*

At the first sign of redness, irritation, scratching or rubbing of the ears, clean your pet's ears.

Essential oils applied around the base of the ear can help treat an ear infection and/or prevent an infection. Never pour essential oils directly into the ear canal. Lavender, Geranium, Frankincense, Myrrh and Arborvitae are all essential oils that kill infection-causing bacteria and yeast and help to ease any discomfort your pet may be feeling as a result of an ear infection. For chronic ear infections make sure to apply essential oils extending from the base of the ear down the side of the neck.

Ailments, Conditions, and Other Issues

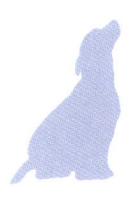

FOR DOGS

Apply 1 drop each Geranium, Lavender, and Myrrh in 1 tsp. carrier oil around the base of the ear- front and back, on the outside only, 2–3 times daily. For additional support, add 1 drop each Frankincense and Arborvitae to the above oils in 2 tsp. carrier oil.

Diffuse Protective Blend daily for 20–30 minutes 2–3 times daily.

Support the immune system with a healthy diet supplemented with Omega-3 and a probiotic.

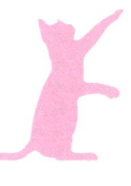

FOR CATS

Apply 1 drop each Geranium, Lavender, and Myrrh in 2 tsp. carrier oil around the base of the ear- front and back, on the outside only, 2–3 times daily. For additional support, add 1 drop each Frankincense and Arborvitae in 4 tsp. carrier oil.

Diffuse Protective Blend daily for 20 - 30 minutes 2–3 times daily.

Support the immune system with a healthy diet supplemented with Omega-3 and a probiotic.

EAR MITES

Ear Mites in cats are parasites that live only in the ear canals and are highly contagious between cats. Ear mites are diagnosed with a microscopic exam performed by your veterinarian. Most commonly, ear mites cause black debris in the ears which lead to scratching and irritation. Lavender, Geranium, Outdoor Blend, and Rosemary are a good complement to traditional treatment and are beneficial in helping to eliminate ear mites. Essential oils reduce itch and relieve irritation in the ear. **Never** pour essential oils directly into the ear canal.

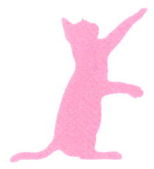

FOR CATS

Clean your cats ears weekly (See Ear Cleaning).

Mix 1 drop each of Lavender, Geranium, Outdoor Blend and Rosemary in 4 tsp. of carrier oil and apply the mixture daily around the base of your cat's ears. Also apply the mixture at the very tips of the ear daily using a finger or cotton swab. Never pour essential oils directly into the ear canal.

Note: When using essential oils for cats or for any condition which persists or worsens, contact your veterinarian.

Ailments, Conditions, and Other Issues

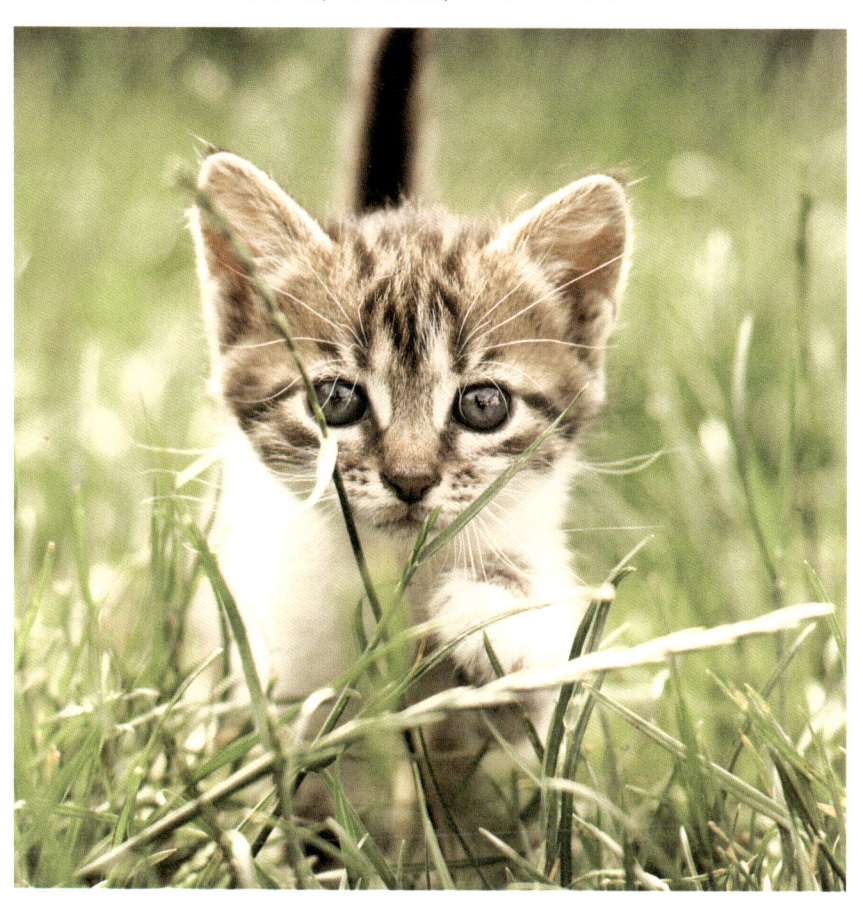

"Time spent with cats is never wasted."

-Sigmund Freud

EMOTIONAL CONNECTION WITH THE ORGANS OF THE BODY

Emotions are how we and our pets respond to our feelings. Each emotional response is paralleled by a biological response and psychological process. Traditional Chinese medicine views seven emotions including joy, anger, anxiety, grief, pensiveness, fear and fright and each affects the health of an organ. Historically, Greek medicine, the root of traditional western medicine, also viewed that emotions affect the health of the organs.

Traditional Chinese medicine, which has been practiced for more than five thousand years, has a central principle that classifies five major organ system pairs that are each associated with a particular emotion. The liver and gallbladder are associated with anger, the heart and small intestine are associated with joy, the spleen and stomach are associated with over-thinking or pensiveness, the lungs and large intestine are associated with grief, and the kidney and bladder are associated with fear.

Joy
Joy is an emotion of deep contentment and is connected to the heart, according to traditional Chinese medicine. Feelings of overexcitement, excess joy can lead to agitation, insomnia, fever and heart palpitations.

Anger
Anger is an emotion that is associated with resentment, frustration, irritability and rage. Chinese medicine asserts that this emotion is stored in the liver and gallbladder, which produce and store bile, respectively. This anger can affect many biological processes that decrease energy and cause dizziness and high blood pressure.

Ailments, Conditions, and Other Issues

Anxiety

Anxiety is an emotion of excessive worry that can affect the lungs and large intestine. Anxiety may result in shortness of breath, diarrhea and ulcerative colitis, an inflammation of the large intestine. The consequences being low energy due to decreased levels of oxygen and lack of proper nutrition.

Grief

Grief creates disharmony in the lungs and blocks energy from circulating throughout the body. Grief can destroy the will to live and result in respiratory conditions.

Pensiveness

Pensiveness is an emotion of overthinking. Pensiveness affects the spleen and can cause fatigue, lethargy and inability to concentrate. It can disrupt normal digestion and lead to gas, distention and bloating.

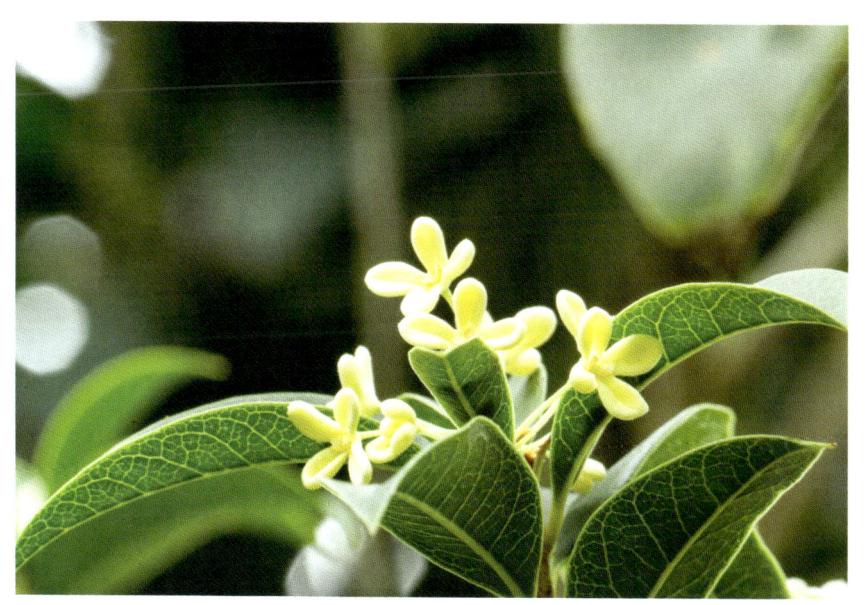

Osmanthus found in a grounding blend

Fear
Fear is an emotion that can cause disharmony in the kidneys and bladder causing involuntary urination. According to Greek Medicine, extreme fear can lead to incontinence.

Fright
Fright is an emotion of shock and panic due to something sudden or unexpected. Fright initially affects the heart, and chronic fright can affect the kidneys.

The connection between the organs and emotions may play a role in your pet's health and in the ability to heal. For example, grief is associated with the lungs and large intestine. Therefore, a pet who has lost a human companion or another pet in the household may benefit from using oils that support these organs. On the other hand, aiding a pet with a physical ailment may include attending to the emotions that are associated with the affected organ system. For example, a pet with Liver disease may be helped by using oils that decrease anger such as Geranium.

Overall health is a combination of emotional and physical wellbeing and balance. The goal of healing is to consider both the state of body and mind. The complexity and diverse chemistry of essential oils offers us the ability to support the entire being and to take a holistic approach in caring for our pets.

FELINE ACNE

Cats often develop acne on their chins and around their lips. Often this is due to plastic bowls or toys, food allergies and contact allergies to chemicals such as fragrances, cleaning products and laundry products (See Allergies, Green Cleaning). Addressing any underlying causes and feeding a high quality diet is crucial for maintaining overall health. Administer a probiotic supplement to support the immune system. We recommend you have your pet tested for environmental and food allergies, change to stainless steel, glass or ceramic bowls and switch to natural cleaning products. Wash your cat's chin daily with Gentle Cleanser, apply Lavender and/or Myrrh essential oils and a Healing Salve daily. If the breakouts persist, consider changing your cat's diet (See Nutrition) and see your veterinarian.

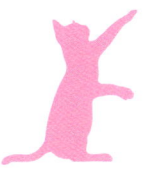

FOR CATS

Wash your cat's chin daily with Gentle Cleanser.

Apply 1 drop Lavender and/or Myrrh in 2 tsp. carrier oil and apply to affected area twice daily.

Feed your cat a high quality diet supplemented with Omega-3 and probiotics.

Gentle Cleanser

Ingredients
4 oz. Castile soap or unscented natural foaming soap
2 drops Roman Chamomile Essential Oil
2 drops Lavender Essential Oil
Glass or Plastic Container*

Instructions
Add essential oils to glass or plastic container. Top with soap. Shake the bottle well before use. Lather and rinse well.

Healing Salve

Ingredients
8 oz. Cold-Pressed Organic Coconut Oil
1 oz. Beeswax
2 drops Vitamin E (optional)
10 drops Lavender Essential Oil
5 drops Myrrh Essential Oil
3 drops Helichrysum Essential Oil
*Glass Jars , Tin Containers or Plastic Bottle ***

Instructions
Place the coconut oil and beeswax over a double –boiler, and gently warm over low heat until the beeswax melts. Remove from heat and add the essential oils and Vitamin E oil, (if using). Quickly pour the mixture into glass jars, tins, or plastic containers and allow to cool completely. Store salve in a cool location where it will not re-melt and re-solidify. When stored correctly, salve will last for 1–3 years. Yields 8 oz.

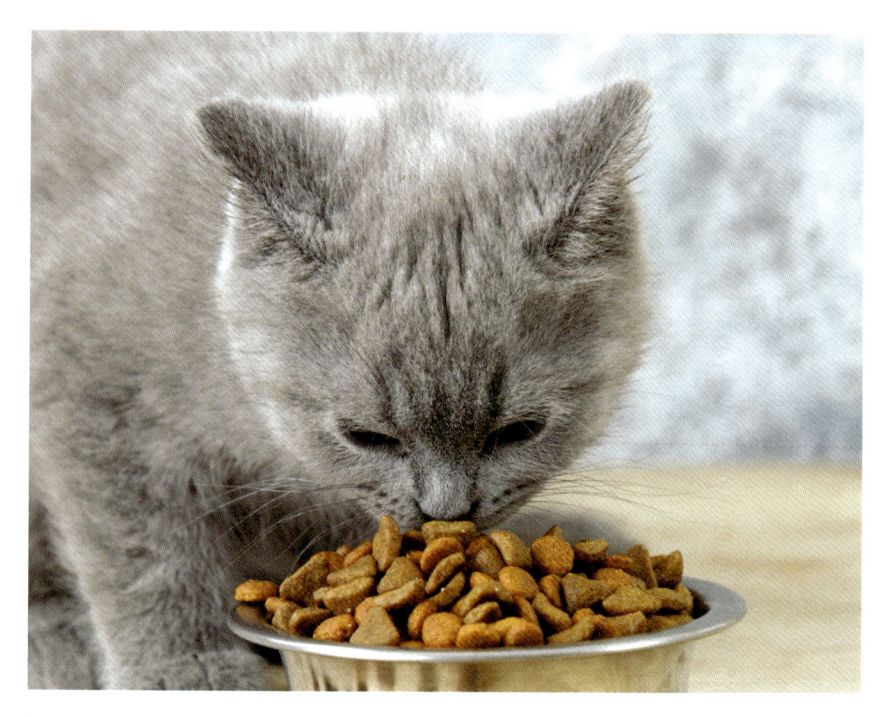

FELINE HERPESVIRUS (FVH-1)

Feline Herpesvirus (FVH-1) or Herpes, also known as Feline Viral Rhinotracheitis (FVR), is the leading cause of conjunctivitis and a major cause of upper respiratory disease in cats (See Respiratory Conditions). In chronic conditions, Feline Herpesvirus may result in scarring of the cornea or permanent dry eye (keratoconjunctivitis sicca, KCS). This highly contagious virus is easily spread among colonies of cats in shelters, outdoor cats, and in multi-cat homes. Saliva and eye and nose discharge of infected cats contains the virus. Therefore, the virus is spread via sneezing, grooming, sharing litter boxes, food and water bowls, and contact with contaminated clothing, bedding or furniture. It may also be spread from a mother to her kittens. To reduce the spread of Herpes, clean and disinfect surfaces using Protective Blend concentrated cleaner (See Green Cleaning). Launder contaminated bedding, towels and clothing with hot water using Protective Blend laundry detergent.

Signs of Herpes include sneezing, congestion, conjunctivitis, eye and nasal discharge, eye ulcers, fever, lethargy and decreased appetite. Infected cats suffer from a weakened immune system, making them susceptible to secondary infections. An infected cat shows signs of infection 2–5 days after exposure and can transmit the virus during this time and for up to 3 weeks after developing symptoms. Once infected with Herpes, a cat becomes a lifelong carrier of the virus meaning the virus remains in the cat's body for his or her entire life. Infected cats with or without symptoms, may pass the virus to other cats. Infected cats my suffer periodic flare ups throughout their lives as a result of stress, changes in environment or changes in schedule (See Anxiety and Stress, Grief).

Protect your cat by minimizing contact with other cats, and by keeping your cat(s) indoors. When introducing a new cat to your home, keep him or her isolated from other cats in the home for two weeks and observe for any signs of illness.

There is no cure for Herpes. The goal of treatment is to reduce the severity and frequency of recurrent illness. Herpes and secondary infections are treated with antibiotics, eye medication and oral antiviral medication. An amino acid, L-lysine, has been shown to help alleviate signs of illness and keep the virus in a latent or quiet state. Cats who carry Herpes may continue to take L-lysine supplements throughout their lives to reduce Herpes outbreaks. Consult your veterinarian to discuss vaccinating against Feline Herpesvirus.

Feed a high quality diet supplemented with Omega-3 and probiotics. Probiotics have been proven to support the immune system, reduce stress and decrease the length of time a cat is sick. Additionally, essential oils may support the immune system, speed recovery and support overall well-being.

A number of essential oils are supportive to the immune system and have anti-viral properties. These oils will help your cat to handle any secondary infections and any complications that may occur. We suggest applying a combination of Thyme, Melissa, Copaiba, Geranium, and Frankincense daily. Diffuse a combination of Protective Blend, Copaiba and Frankincense to purify the air supporting your cat and any other cats in the household. Stress plays a role in healing and suppresses the immune system. Apply and diffuse one of the following calming essential oils: Restful Blend, Renewing Blend, or Grounding Blend. In a multi-cat household, support all of your cats with daily application of Frankincense and Copaiba (See Longevity: A Long and Healthy Life).

Ailments, Conditions, and Other Issues

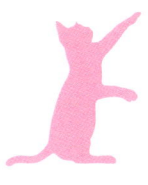

FOR CATS

Infected Cats: Apply 1 drop each Thyme, Melissa, Copaiba, Geranium, and Frankincense in 2 tsp. carrier oil for cats in 4 tsp. carrier for kittens twice daily.

Diffuse Protective Blend or Copaiba and Frankincense for 20–30 minutes 2–3 times daily.

Diffuse Restful Blend, Renewing Blend, or Grounding Blend for 20–30 minutes 2–3 times daily.

Feed a high quality diet supplemented with Omega-3 and probiotics.

Non-infected cats or kittens in a multi-cat household: Apply 1 drop each Copaiba and Frankincense in 2 tsp. carrier oil for cats in 4 tsp. carrier for kittens twice daily.

Feed a high quality diet supplemented with Omega-3 and probiotics.

"Never try to outstubborn a cat."

-Robert A. Heinlein

FELINE IMMUNODEFICIENCY VIRUS

Feline Immunodeficiency Virus (FIV), also known as feline AIDS, is a serious viral disease that affects cats and suppresses their immune system. FIV-infected cats are found worldwide, but the prevalence of infection varies greatly. In the United States, approximately 1.5 - 3 percent of healthy cats are infected with FIV. Infected cats may harbor this disease with no signs of illness for several years.

Feline Immunodeficiency Virus (FIV) is primarily spread through bite wounds. The most common population of cats infected with FIV are outdoor males who typically fight to defend territory and to acquire females. This is the perfect reason to keep your cat indoors. Casual contact, such as grooming, sharing food and water bowls and litter boxes, among cats who live together is not likely to spread this disease.

FIV is characterized by chronic and recurrent infections. Cats are exposed to bacteria, viruses, and fungal organisms all the time. Since FIV attacks the immune system, an infected cat may suffer severe illness from these common everyday microbes. Signs of FIV include anemia, fever, weight loss, poor coat, decreased appetite, inflammation of the mouth and gums, non-healing wounds, diarrhea, sneezing, neurologic signs and changes in behavior (See Diarrhea and Vomiting, Seizures).

Veterinary hospitals and shelters commonly test for FIV, if any new kittens or cats are brought into the home or in any cat that suddenly becomes ill. There is no direct treatment for this virus, and secondary infections and illnesses, which may affect multiple organ systems throughout the body, need to be addressed as they occur. If secondary infections are well managed, these cats may live normal lifespans. Using essential oils will support a healthy immune system so that your cat is better able to combat any possible secondary infections and resulting symptoms.

Ailments, Conditions, and Other Issues

Although vaccination is available, limit exposure to outdoor and feral cats. See your veterinarian at least twice annually to closely monitor your cat's weight and perform routine annual diagnostic testing. Spay and neuter your cat, keep him or her indoors, and feed a high quality diet supplemented with Omega-3 and probiotics.

A number of essential oils are supportive to the immune system and have anti-viral properties. These oils will help your cat to handle any secondary infections and any complications that may occur. We suggest applying a combination of Thyme, Melissa, Copaiba, Geranium, and Frankincense daily. Diffuse a combination of Protective Blend, Copaiba and Frankincense to purify the air supporting your cat and any other cats in the household. Stress plays a role in healing and suppresses the immune system. Apply and diffuse one of the following calming essential oils: Restful Blend, Renewing Blend, or Grounding Blend. In a multi-cat household, support all of your cats with daily application of Frankincense and Copaiba (See Longevity: A Long and Healthy Life).

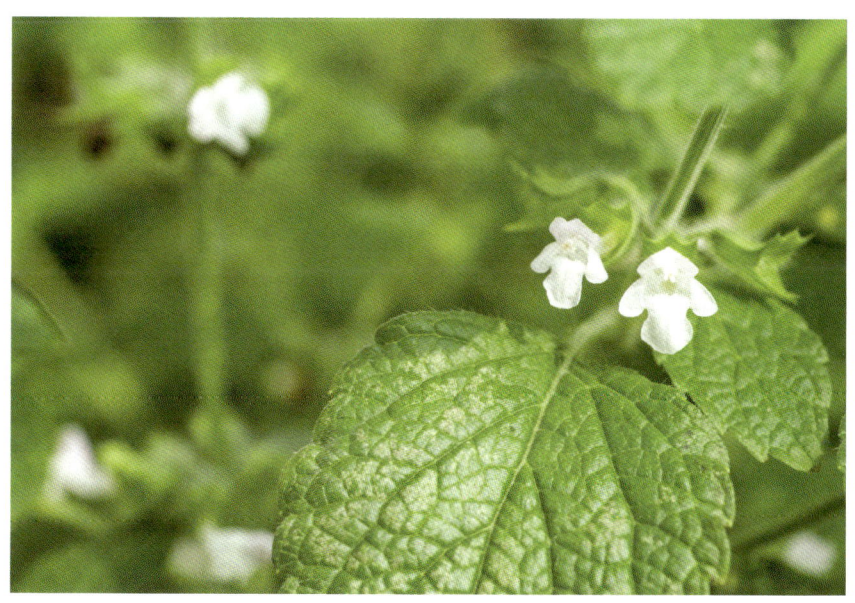

Melissa

"It is impossible to keep a straight face in the presence of one or more kittens."

-Cynthia E. Varnado

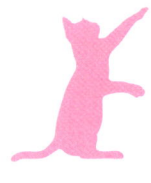

FOR CATS

For infected cats: Apply 1 drop each Thyme, Melissa, Copaiba, Geranium, and Frankincense in 2 tsp carrier oil for cats in 4 tsp carrier for kittens twice daily.

Diffuse Protective Blend or Copaiba and Frankincense for 20–30 minutes 2–3 times daily.

Diffuse Restful Blend, Renewing Blend, or Grounding Blend for 20–30 minutes 2–3 times daily.

Feed a high quality diet supplemented with Omega-3 and probiotics.

For non-infected cats or kittens in a multi-cat household:
Apply 1 drop each Copaiba and Frankincense in 2 tsp carrier oil for cats in 4 tsp carrier for kittens twice daily.

Feed a high quality diet supplemented with Omega-3 and probiotics.

Ailments, Conditions, and Other Issues

FELINE LEUKEMIA VIRUS

Feline Leukemia Virus (FeLV) is a serious viral disease that affects cats and suppresses their immune system. It is one of the most common infectious diseases in cats, affecting between 2–3% of all cats in the United States. Veterinary hospitals and shelters commonly test new kittens and any newly acquired cat for FeLV.

Infected cats, may harbor this virus with no signs of illness for several years and remain symptom free. In other cats, FeLV becomes active, and the cat will become ill. FeLV infects the bone marrow, often causes anemia, suppresses the immune system and may lead to autoimmune disease. FeLV can cause sterility and lead to stillbirths and is the leading cause of cancer in cats (See Cancer). Signs of FeLV include pale gums, fever, weight loss, lethargy, diarrhea, and weakness (See Diarrhea and Vomiting, Anorexia and Loss of Appetite). Due to a suppressed immune system, an infected cat may suffer severe illness from common everyday bacteria, viruses and fungal organisms. There is no direct treatment for this virus and no cure. Secondary infections and illnesses are treated as they may occur. Essential oils can support the immune system and help address infections and illnesses due to this virus.

This disease is highly contagious and is transmitted via saliva, urine and blood, in utero and by nursing. The virus is spread from cat to cat by grooming, sharing food and water bowls and litter boxes (See Green Cleaning). In a multi-cat household, preventing the spread of infection may be challenging. An FeLV vaccination is available and we suggest speaking to your veterinarian about immunizing your cat(s). We advise keeping a FeLV positive cat away from negative cats as much as possible and using essential oils to keep your feline household healthy.

Due to the severity of this disease and the fact that there is no cure, we suggest that you spay or neuter your cat. Keep him or her indoors limiting your cat's exposure to outdoor or feral cats.

Feed your a high quality diet supplemented with Omega-3 and probiotics.

A number of essential oils are supportive to the immune system and have anti-viral properties. These oils will help your to cat to handle any secondary infections and any complications that may occur. We suggest applying a combination of Thyme, Melissa, Copaiba, Geranium, and Frankincense daily. Diffuse a combination of Protective Blend, Copaiba and Frankincense to purify the air supporting your cat and any other cats in the household. Stress plays a role in healing and suppresses the immune system. Apply and diffuse one of the following calming essential oils: Restful Blend, Renewing Blend, or Grounding Blend. In a multi-cat household, support all of your cats with daily application of Frankincense and Copaiba (See Longevity: A Long and Healthy Life).

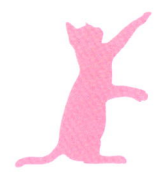

FOR CATS

For infected cats: Apply 1 drop each Thyme, Melissa, Copaiba, Geranium, and Frankincense in 2 tsp carrier oil for cats in 4 tsp carrier for kittens twice daily.

Diffuse Protective Blend or Copaiba and Frankincense for 20–30 minutes 2–3 times daily.

Diffuse Restful Blend, Renewing Blend, or Grounding Blend for 20–30 minutes 2–3 times daily.

Feed a high quality diet supplemented with Omega-3 and probiotics.

For non-infected cats or kittens in a multi-cat household:
Apply 1 drop each Copaiba and Frankincense in 2 tsp carrier oil for cats in 4 tsp carrier for kittens twice daily.

Feed a high quality diet supplemented with Omega-3 and probiotics.

Ailments, Conditions, and Other Issues

FIRST AID

Accidents happen, and it is best to be prepared by keeping a basic first aid kit for the pets in your household. Put together a well-provisioned first aid kit containing basic items and essential oils so that you will be ready for a medical emergency if one arises. We suggest making a second first that can be kept in the car and will travel with you, as accidents don't only happen at home. An easy kit can be prepared in an insulated lunch bag, which will keep all the items dry and protected. Always keep contact information for your vet, emergency hospital and animal poison control center handy.

Some general supplies and necessities to include in your kit include, a copy of SpOIL Your Pet, wash cloth, gauze, tape, small scissors, tweezers, a small flashlight, roll-on bottles, clean socks to cover a bandage and disposable gloves. Additional items to include are bottled water, saline solution, apple cider vinegar, honey or maple syrup, cornstarch, aloe vera gel, Gentle Cleanser, Healing Salve, carrier oil and essential oils.

The following selection of essential oils will be useful in a number of situations: Lavender, Frankincense, Myrrh, Helichrysum, Peppermint, Massage Blend, Protective Blend, Digestive Blend, Restful Blend and Grounding Blend. Attend to cuts and scrapes with Myrrh, Helichrysum, Frankincense, and Lavender. Address any digestive upset or motion sickness with Digestive Blend and Lavender. Manage sore muscles after a long walk or hike with Frankincense and Massage Blend. Initiate care for heat stroke with Peppermint, Frankincense and Massage Blend. Emergencies are stressful for both your pet and you maintain a sense of calm with Restful Blend and Grounding Blend. Protective Blend is supportive to the immune system and partners well with any essential oil. It complements other oils used in any incident.

Refer to specific sections of this book for detailed information and clear instructions on what to do in various situations.

FLEAS, TICKS, AND MOSQUITOES

Fleas, ticks and mosquitoes carry a number of diseases and parasites. Some of these are not only dangerous to your pets, but also to you and your family. The most common consequences of flea, tick and mosquito bites include Heartworm disease (from mosquitoes), Bartonella/Cat Scratch Fever (from fleas and ticks), Tapeworms (from fleas) and Lyme disease (from ticks). (See Heartworm Disease, Bartonella,, Tick-Borne Diseases, Worms).

These parasites are present across much of the United States and around the world and are found in many different environments and climates. Fleas, ticks and mosquitoes can survive all year round despite changes in the seasons.

Fleas, in particular, can be very difficult to rid from the home. Thus, prevention is the best way to avoid the many possible consequences of fleas, ticks and mosquitoes. Geranium, Thyme, Arborvitae or Outdoor Blend repel insects, fleas, and ticks effectively for several hours. Pure essential oils are perfectly safe for you, your children and your pets.

If fleas or ticks have invaded your home, a combination approach is most effective. Treat your home with a natural flea bomb. Clean your home with Protective Blend cleaner concentrate, launder bedding with Protective Blend laundry detergent and diffuse Cleansing Blend or Protective Blend in your home. Bathe and spray pets with Flea and Tick Repellant Shampoo and Spray effective against pests.

Ailments, Conditions, and Other Issues

FOR DOGS & CATS

Fleas: For prevention, dilute Outdoor Blend 1:1 with water in a glass spray bottle or use a pre-diluted Outdoor Blend Spray. For further protection, use Flea and Tick Repellant Spray. Apply by spraying your hands and apply to your pet's entire body, including torso, legs and underside 2–3 times daily. Be careful to avoid the eyes.

Prepare a Do-It-Yourself Homemade Flea and Tick Collar.

If fleas have invaded your home, a combination approach is most effective:

Treat your home with a Natural Flea Bomb.

Clean your home with Protective Blend cleaner concentrate.

Launder bedding with Protective Blend laundry detergent.

Diffuse Cleansing Blend or Protective Blend in your home.

Bathe pets with Flea and Tick Repellant Shampoo effective against pests.

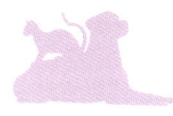

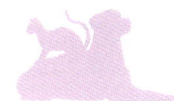

Continue these steps to prevent pests all year round.

FOR DOGS & CATS

Ticks: For prevention, dilute Cleansing Blend, or Outdoor Blend 1:1 with water in a glass spray bottle or use a pre-diluted Outdoor Blend Spray. Add to either of these mixtures 5 drops each Geranium and Thyme per 30ml (1 oz.). Shake well and apply by spraying your hands and apply to your pet's entire body, including torso, legs and underside 2–3 times daily. Be careful to avoid the eyes.

Bathe with Flea and Tick Repellant Shampoo.

Continue these steps to prevent pests all year round.

SpOil Your Pet

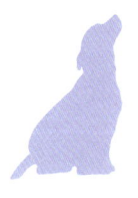

FOR DOGS

Flea, Mosquito, and Tick Bites: Apply 1 drop each Lavender, Massage Blend, and Myrrh in 1 tsp. carrier oil directly to Flea, Mosquito, or Tick bites 3–4 times daily for as long as needed.

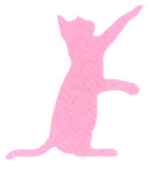

FOR CATS

Flea, Mosquito, and Tick Bites: Apply 1 drop each Lavender and Myrrh directly in 2 tsp. carrier oil directly to Flea, Mosquito, or Tick bites 3–4 times daily for as long as needed.

Call your veterinarian if needed.

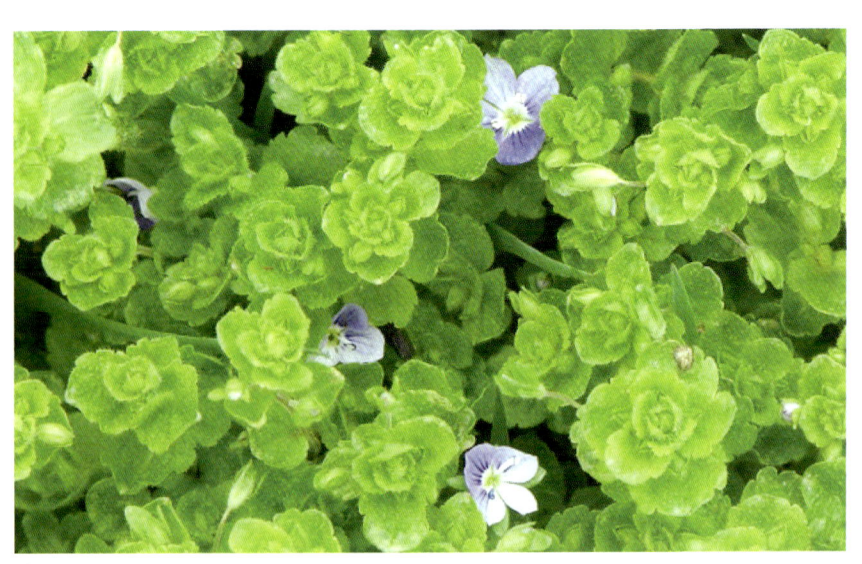

Thyme

Natural Flea Bomb

Ingredients
10 drops Black Pepper Essential Oil
10 drops Oregano Essential Oil
10 drops Orange Essential Oil
10 drops Peppermint Essential Oil
10 drops Cleansing Essential Oil Blend (to be used after "flea bombing" the house)

Instructions
Add the essential oils to a water diffuser or in an empty bottle for a nebulizer diffuser. Open all the interior doors in your home and place the diffuser in the most central location possible. If there is a heavy infestation in more than one room you will need to treat each room individually. Turn your diffuser on to maximum output and use a continuous diffusion for 2–3 hours. Leave your home during this time and take your pets with you if possible. If you are not able to take your pets, try to keep them in a separate room away from the diffuser. Upon returning home, open all the windows in your home. Diffuse Cleansing Blend for another 1–2 hours.

Now it is time to vacuum everywhere! Move furniture and vacuum behind it and under it. Vacuum the furniture, too. Empty the vacuum when you are finished, and discard any contents outside of your home.

Flea & Tick Repellent Shampoo or Spray

Ingredients
8 oz. Natural Shampoo Base or Water
4 drops Clary Sage Essential Oil
2 drops Cleansing Essential Oil Blend
5 drops Repellant Essential Oil Blend
8 drops Peppermint Essential Oil
4 drops Lemon Essential Oil
2 drops Geranium Essential Oil
2 drops Eucalyptus Essential Oil

3 drops Lavender Essential Oil
2 drops Myrrh Essential Oil
2 drops Thyme Essential Oil
Glass or Plastic Bottle*

Instructions:

Add essential oils to an empty glass or plastic bottle. Top with water. Shake the bottle well before use. Spray your pet, bedding and yourself!

Homemade Flea and Tick Collar

Ingredients

5 drops Eucalyptus Essential Oil
5 drops Geranium Essential oil
5 drops Thyme Essential Oil
5 drops Lemongrass Essential Oil
5 drops Repellant Essential Oil Blend
4 oz. distilled water
Glass or Plastic Container*

For puppies younger than 4 months or for dogs weighing less than 15 pounds, use 2 drops of each recommended essential oil in 8 oz. of distilled water.

For cats, use 1 drop each Arborvitae, Geranium, Thyme, Lemongrass, and Repellant Blend in 8 oz. of distilled water.

Instructions

Mix distilled water with the essential oils in a glass or plastic container. Soak a nylon/cloth collar in the solution for 20 minutes.

Remove collar and allow it to dry thoroughly before placing it on your pet.

Re-soak the collar every two weeks or more frequently as needed.

GASTRIC ULCERS

The most common cause of gastric ulceration is the administration of Non-Steroidal Anti-Inflammatory Drugs (NSAID's). This class of medication is used to treat pain and reduce inflammation. Medications in this class include Tylenol, Aspirin, Motrin, and Aleve. If your pet needs to take a non-steroidal medication, your veterinarian will prescribe one tested in dogs and cats and safe for their use. Do not use medications designated for human consumption on your pets.

Gastric upset, irritation, bleeding and ulcers are more likely to develop when over-the-counter medications are used in high doses or for extended periods of time. Never medicate your pet without consulting your veterinarian. The use of non-steroidal medications (NSAID's) should be closely monitored by your veterinarian with blood work and frequent visits.

If your pet needs a non-steroidal medication, protect your pet's gastrointestinal system from damage with essential oils. The use of anti-inflammatory essential oils may allow you to decrease the amount of medication your pet is taking.

For dogs, apply a combination of Digestive Blend, Myrrh, Copaiba and Lavender daily. This will support and calm the digestive system. For immune support, diffuse Protective Blend. Give your dog a probiotic supplement to further support the gastrointestinal system.

For cats, apply a combination of Digestive Blend, Myrrh, Copaiba and Lavender daily, and add Lavender and/or Digestive Blend to the litter box (See Recipes: Litter Box Power). For immune support, diffuse Protective Blend. Give your cat a probiotic supplement to further support the gastrointestinal system.

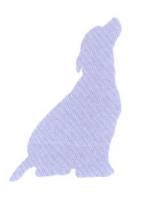

FOR DOGS

Apply 1 drop each Digestive Blend, Lavender, Copiaba and Myrrh in 2 tsp. carrier oil twice daily.

Diffuse Protective Blend for at least 20–30 minutes 2–3 times daily.

Continue probiotic supplements.

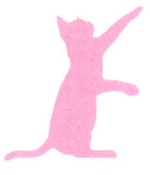

FOR CATS

Apply 1 drop each Digestive Blend, Lavender, Copaiba and Myrrh in 4 tsp. carrier oil twice daily.

Add Lavender and/or Digestive Blend to the litter box (See Recipes: Litter Box Power).

Diffuse Protective Blend for at least 20–30 minutes 2–3 times daily.

Continue probiotic supplements.

"Dogs lives are too short. Thier only fault, really."

- Agnes Sligh Turnbull

GRIEF AND LOSS

There are many types of loss that we and our pets can experience throughout our lives from loss of a companion pet, to loss of an owner or caretaker or other family member or friend. Pets, like people, mourn the loss of a loved one and may become depressed and sad.

It is well documented that the loss of a companion pet or animal can be difficult for the remaining dog or cat in the household. Our four legged companions not only are responding to their own loss but also perceive and sense our loss and the feeling of grief in the home. One of the most drastic changes, when one pet in a multi-pet household dies, is the change in the structure of the 'pack' hierarchy. Dogs and cats have very well defined social roles, with leaders and followers. Without your/their companion, the remaining pet's role may be ill-defined.

Loss of an owner or caretaker can also be traumatic for our pets. Animals are very sensitive and emotional. They become very attached and reliant on us not only for their basic needs like food and care but affection and love.

You may notice both physical and behavioral changes in response to a loss. Such as, avoiding social interaction, hiding or segregating himself or herself from the family, a change in play habits and decreased desire to go outside or walk. Some dogs may pace or even look like they are 'searching' for their lost loved one. Pets may wait at the door or sleep at the base of a bed. Some dogs and cats may vocalize excessively, crying out for their companion or owner. Physically, a change in appetite, which can lead to weight loss or gain, can also occur. Grooming habits may change in cats and urination and bathroom habits may be altered in both dogs and cats.

As the saying goes "Time Heals All Wounds". Remember that we all mourn in our own way and that includes pets. So, be patient and loving and allow your pet the time and space that it needs to heal.

There are easy steps you can take to ease your pet's grief. Among them, diffuse or apply essential oils which can help shift the emotional environment of your home.

How to Help Your Grieving Pet

1. Engage your dog or cat in a new activity. Positive training is a beneficial way to help your pet learn its new position in the family, and this bond and communication make it easy for the pet to look to you for leadership.

2. A training class that uses positive methods or private lessons from a trainer may help you to learn the skills you'll need to help your pet shift it's focus from loss to enthusiasm.

3. Increasing the activities your dog or cat loves to do also helps a grieving dog or cat to cope. Investing time with your other pet(s), will also help you process your emotions. For example, a dog that loves to play fetch at the park might benefit from a few more fetch sessions. Simple things like getting to ride in the car while you run errands, extra brushing time, a new squeaky toy, or for a cat playing with a laser light or fishing rod toy, may captivate your pet's attention and make them feel loved. Even just a few more minutes of play time or attention can help your dog or cat adjust to life without it's companion, and may make you feel better too!

4. Touch between a human and a pet has therapeutic benefits for both species. In humans, petting a dog or cat can trigger the release of the bonding hormone oxytocin. Oxytocin acts as a chemical messenger in the brain and has been shown to be important in human feelings including trust, safety and reassurance. Feeling your pet's fur can also lower your heart rate and blood pressure.

Combining petting, with the application of essential oils further enhances the time you will spend with your pet and will foster healing for you both. Essential oils will be absorbed through the coat and skin and will promote feelings of peace and comfort.

5. The olfactory system includes all physical organs or cells relating to, or contributing to, the sense of smell. When we inhale through the nose, airborne molecules interact with the olfactory organs and, almost immediately, the brain. Diffusing essential oils can help shift the emotional environment of your home. Inhaled essential oils can affect the body through several systems and pathways. During inhalation, odor molecules travel through the nose and affect the brain through a variety of receptor sites, one of which is the limbic system, which is commonly referred to as the "emotional brain." Secondly, molecules inhaled through the nose are carried to the lungs and interact with the respiratory system.

In ancient cultures, the emotion of grief is concentrated in the sinuses and lungs. Marjoram and Cypress are healing to the heart and respiratory system and help our pets and us to process various emotions. This enables us to let that emotion go. Some of our favorite essential oils for emotional support are Comforting Blend, Reassuring Blend, Bergamot, Cedarwood, Cypress, Marjoram, Centering Blend, Restful Blend and Uplifting Blend. The oils may be diffused individually or in combination. Here are a few suggestions: 2–3 drops each Comforting Blend and Cedarwood or 2 drops each Reassuring Blend, Cypress, and Marjoram in a diffuser that holds 240 ml or 1 cup of water.

Diffusing essential oils is especially helpful when a pet is avoiding human interaction. Other possible ways to introduce essential oils to your pet is by placing a few drops of essential oil on a stuffed toy or pet bed, which passively exposes your pet to the healing benefits of essential oils.

Both diffusing and topical application of essential oils act powerfully to affect your pet's physical and emotional state as well as your own.

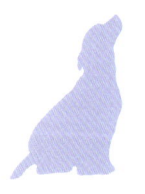

FOR DOGS

Apply 1 drop each Comforting Blend, Reassuring Blend, Cypress and Marjoram in 1 tsp. carrier oil 2–3 times daily.

Diffuse 2–3 drops each Comforting Blend and Cedarwood or 2 drops each Reassuring Blend, Cypress, and Marjoram in a diffuser that holds 240 ml or 1 cup of water.

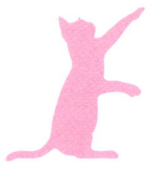

FOR CATS

Apply 1 drop each Comforting Blend, Reassuring Blend, Cypress and Marjoram in 2 tsp. carrier oil 2–3 times daily.

Diffuse 2–3 drops each Comforting Blend and Cedarwood or 2 drops each Reassuring Blend, Cypress, and Marjoram in a diffuser that holds 240 ml or 1 cup of water.

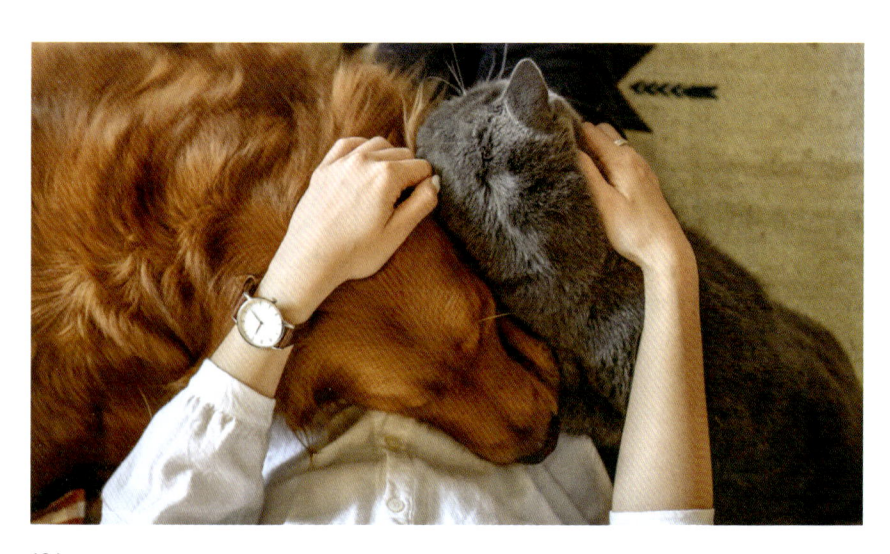

GROOMING AND BASIC PET CARE

Caring for your pet helps to create and sustain a special bond between you and your pet which is strengthened by spending time together. Grooming is both enjoyable for you and your pet.
To keep your pet's skin and coat healthy and to reduce shedding, feed your pet a high quality diet supplemented with Omega-3 and probiotics. A shiny and silky coat is an indicator of optimal health.

Brushing your pet helps to distribute the natural oils and remove dry dead skin cells and hair. Brush your dog or cat at least three times weekly to maintain a healthy, unknotted coat. Longer haired dogs and cats and those cats prone to hair balls (See Hairballs) benefit from more frequent brushing up to daily. We recommend a slicker brush and a wide-toothed comb for most grooming needs, using caution on the face and around the eyes. Speak with your groomer or veterinarian for individual advice.

Dogs who are considered to be non-shedding or hypoallergenic such as poodles, Maltese, Shih-Tzu, Bichon Frise, and Terriers, need to be professionally groomed every 3–8 weeks, on average. Hypoallergenic breeds have hair which continually grows and needs to be trimmed regularly. If your pet is matted or has large knots in their coat, see your groomer or veterinarian for assistance. Do not attempt to cut your own dog's hair, since the risk of injury to your pet is high. Leave scissoring or clipping your pet to a professional.

We can all appreciate a clean pet, yet bathing too frequently can dry your dog's skin and lead to knots and mats. Cats generally do not accept bathing well, and most cats keep themselves clean without getting a bath for their entire lives. It is very important to comb and/or brush your dog after bathing to prevent the hair from forming knots which may then develop into larger mats. Repeated bathing without proper brushing and combing leads to matting of the coat. Bathing frequently will also remove the monthly liquid flea and tick preventatives, thereby lessening your dog's protection. Bathe your dog with Soothing Skin Shampoo (See recipe below) every 2–4 weeks unless directed by your veterinarian for a medical reason. Following every bath, clean your dog's ears to prevent infection (see Ear Cleaning and Ear Infections). Routinely, clean your dog's or cat's ears 1–2 times monthly. Increase the frequency of ear cleaning to 2–4 times monthly in warmer, humid weather and after any contact with water such as swimming or exposure to heavy rain.

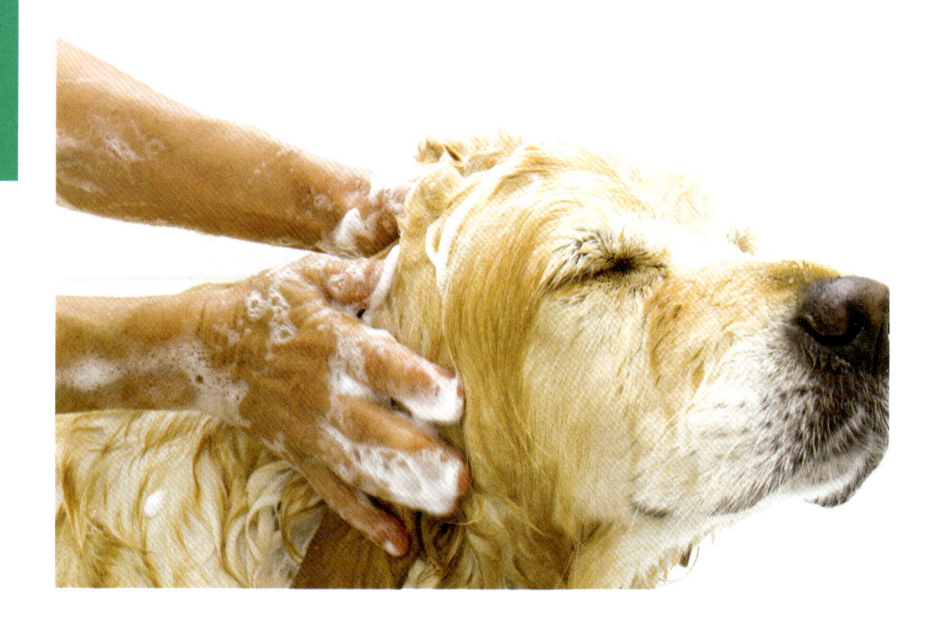

"The most affectionate creature in the world is a wet dog."

- Ambrose Bierce

Ailments, Conditions, and Other Issues

Nail trimming is generally recommended on a monthly basis. Overgrown nails inhibit proper contact of the paws with the ground or floor and place undue tension on the paws and joints which may decrease stability, cause your pet to walk hesitantly and potentially result in a slip or fall. Walking your dog on concrete helps to wear the nails and extend the time between nail trims. Most dogs and cats do not like having their nails trimmed, so you may need to visit your veterinarian or groomer for periodic nail trims. Each nail contains a blood vessel which grows along with the nail. Be careful not to cut the nails too short and cause bleeding and pain. Cutting the nails too short may easily happen if your pet is struggling, moving, shaking or if the nails have grown very long. Alternatively, you may file your pet's nails weekly with a wide nail file or filing block available at beauty supply stores.

Wet dog smell? When our dogs come in from the rain, they often exude a unique odor. Bathing after every outing is neither practical nor advisable. Dry your pet with a towel, and apply the Pet Powder to remove odors naturally. During rainy or snowy months of the year, remove mud and salt by wiping your pet's paws with Gentle Cleanser, cleansing cloths, or a damp towel. If you notice an odor from your pet's eyes, ears, paws or any other part of the body, it may indicate an infection. Contact your veterinarian.

If your dog encounters a skunk, and is unfortunately for you and your dog sprayed, try to remain calm and use our favorite Skunk Remedy to bathe your pet. It is a combination of vinegar, baking soda and Castile soap or natural dish detergent. Do not wet your dog, immediately apply Skunk Remedy to your dog dry. Be careful to avoid the eyes and ears. Massage the Skunk Remedy for 5 minutes and then rinse well and repeat. After towel drying your dog, spray your dog and diffuse cleansing blend as often as needed to remove residual odor. Often, dogs are sprayed in the face and eyes. The skunk's spray may irritate the eyes causing redness, tearing, rubbing and squinting. In this case, see your veterinarian.

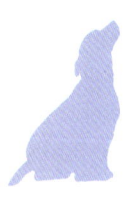

FOR DOGS

Bathe every 2–4 weeks or less. Dry thoroughly.

Clean ears 1–2 times monthly and 2–4 times monthly in warmer, more humid weather.

To remove wet dog smell, apply Pet Powder daily as needed.

To remove skunk odor, do not wet your dog, apply Skunk Remedy massaging for 5 minutes, rinse well and repeat. After towel drying your dog, spray your dog with a solution of 10 drops Cleansing Blend in 1 oz. purified water, as needed.

Diffuse Cleansing Blend to remove odors in your home.

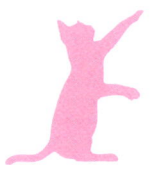

FOR CATS

Brush weekly for short haired cats and 3 times weekly for long haired cats.

Trim nails monthly if possible or have them trimmed by your veterinarian or groomer.

Bathing is best performed by a professional.

Soothing Skin Shampoo

Ingredients
3 oz. Castile soap (available at many health and bulk food stores)
2 oz. Organic unpasteurized, unfiltered Apple Cider Vinegar
1 oz. Vegetable Glycerin
2 oz. Distilled water
3 drops Lavender Essential Oil
3 drops Roman Chamomile Essential Oil
3 drops Myrrh Essential Oil
Optional: *add 1 tsp. ground oatmeal*
Glass or Plastic Bottle*

Instructions
Add essential oils to an empty glass or plastic bottle. Add ground oatmeal (if using). Add the apple cider vinegar, vegetable glycerin, and water to the bottle containing essential oils and oatmeal. Add the castile soap. Shake the bottle well before use.

Skunk Remedy

Ingredients
4 cups Vinegar
1/4 cup Baking Soda
2 tsp. Castile soap or natural dish detergent.

Instructions
Do not wet your dog; immediately apply Skunk Remedy to your dog dry. Be careful to avoid the eyes and ears. Massage the Skunk Remedy for 5 minutes and then rinse well and repeat. After towel drying your dog, spray your dog with a solution of 10 drops Cleansing Blend in 1 oz. purified water, as needed. Diffuse Cleansing Blend to remove odors in your home.

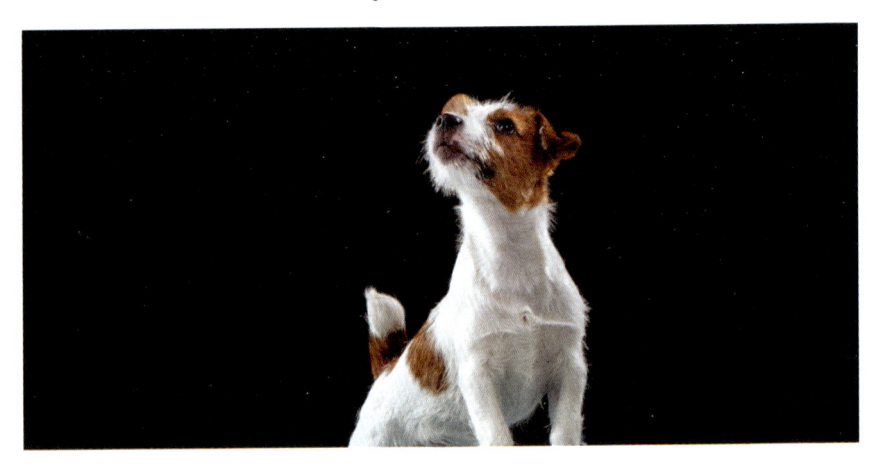

Gentle Cleanser

Ingredients
4 oz. Castile soap or unscented natural foaming soap
2 drops Roman Chamomile Essential Oil
2 drops Lavender Essential Oil
Glass or Plastic Container*

Instructions
Add essential oils to glass or plastic container. Top with soap. Shake the bottle well before use. Lather and rinse well.

Pet Powder

Ingredients
1 Cup Corn Starch
5 drops Lavender Essential Oil
5 drops Geranium Essential Oil
4 drops Eucalyptus Essential Oil
Glass or Plastic Container*

Instructions
Add baking soda to a glass or plastic container. Add essential oils. Mix well, and keep in a small mason jar with several holes in the top. Sprinkle a small amount on your dog and brush him or her. He or she will not only smell great, but repels ticks and other pests.

HAIRBALLS

Contrary to popular belief, hairballs in cats are not normal. Excessive grooming, anxiety, and poor diet are often the cause (See Anxiety and Stress, Obsessive Compulsive Disorder). Cats get hairballs from licking their coats and swallowing hair, which accumulates in the stomach and eventually forms a wad. The accompanying discomfort prompts the cat to vomit the hairball.

Brushing your cat helps to distribute the natural oils and remove dry, dead skin cells and hair. We recommend brushing at least three times weekly or more which will help to reduce the amount of hair ingested (See Grooming and Basic Pet Care).

Feed your cat a high quality diet supplemented with Omega-3 and probiotics and eliminate chemicals in the home (See Green Cleaning). Apply Digestive Blend twice daily to help your cat pass the hairball, and add Digestive Blend to the litter box as described in Litter Box Power (See Recipes: Litter Box Power). Apply or diffuse Lavender or Restful Blend daily to keep your cat calm. Brush your cat 2–3 times weekly to remove excess hair.

In ancient times cats were worshipped as gods; they have not forgotten this.

-Terry Pratchett

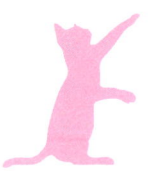

FOR CATS

Apply 1 drop of Digestive Blend in 2 tsp. carrier oil or a pre-diluted roll-on bottle twice daily.

Apply 1 drop of Lavender or Restful Blend in 2 tsp. carrier oil twice daily.

Diffuse Lavender or Restful Blend for 20–30 minutes 2–3 times daily.

Add Digestive Blend to the litter box as described in Litter Box Power.

Brush your cat every 2–3 days to remove excess hair.

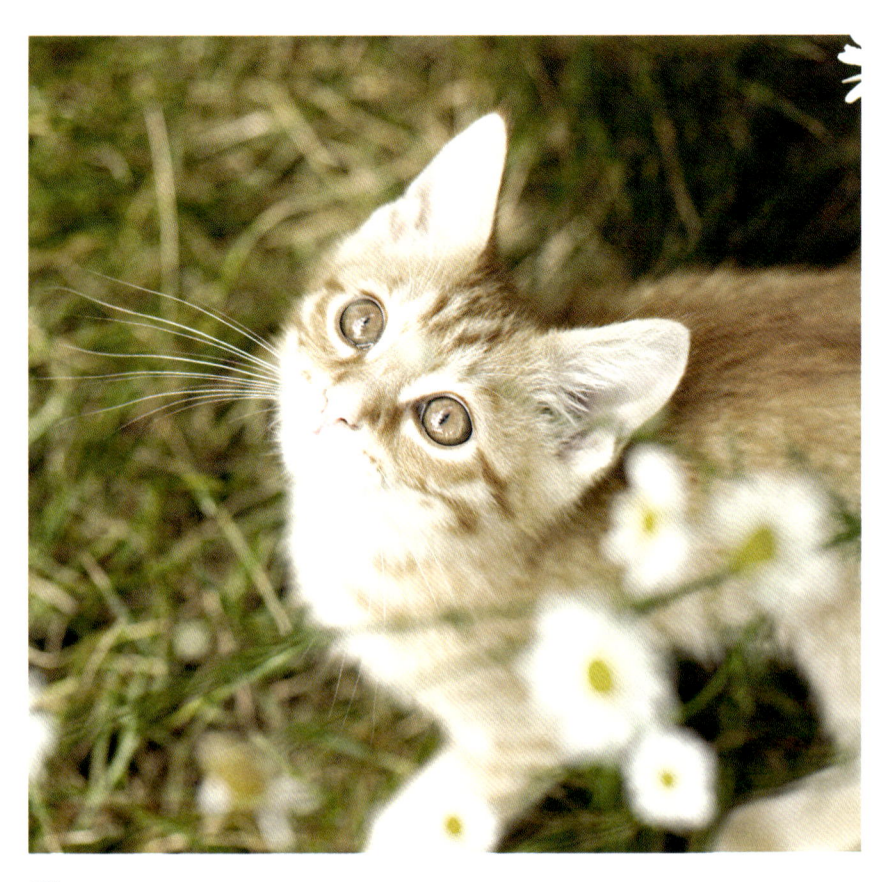

Ailments, Conditions, and Other Issues

HEARTWORM DISEASE

Heartworms are very long worms which live in and around the hearts of dogs and cats and obstruct normal blood flow. Heartworm disease is serious. Dogs and cats with heartworm disease are at risk of death. Heartworms are transmitted by mosquitoes and prevention is critical. (see Fleas, Ticks and Mosquitoes). Although there are reports of essential oil treatments for heartworm disease, we recommend using essential oils as complementary therapy to support a healthy cardiovascular system and immune system. The incidence of heartworm disease in cats is much lower than in dogs, and there is no traditional medical treatment for it in cats (See Organ Support).

Heartworm disease can be found throughout the United States and is more prevalent in areas with high mosquito populations. An annual blood test is recommended for all dogs and cats living in these endemic areas to check for the presence of heartworms. Administer an oral monthly heartworm preventative to your pet as directed by your veterinarian. If your pet tests positive for heartworm and it is found in the early stages, your pet may show no visible signs of illness. As heartworm disease advances, your pet may show signs of lethargy, labored breathing, decreased playfulness and motivation to exercise. Many essential oils have a remarkable ability to both support the immune system and increase one's rate of healing. Some of these same essential oils are also powerful antiseptics. One way these oils fight infection is to stimulate the production of white blood cells, which are part of the body's immune defense. Still other essential oils encourage new cell growth to promote faster healing if your pet gets sick. Lemon essential oil, Rosemary, found in the Protective Blend, and Cypress stimulate the lymphatic system to circulate the blood around the body and remove waste and infection. Copaiba and Ylang Ylang essential oils will help to strengthen and reinforce the cardiovascular system. Frankincense will help support the respiratory system and overall health.

For dogs, support your pet with topical Helichrysum, Oregano (diluted), Copaiba, Ylang Ylang, Frankincense, and Cypress. Oregano is a very powerful anti-parasitic and is recommended here due to the severity of this disease. Add Protective Blend or Lemon to food. Diffuse Protective Blend or Frankincense daily.

For cats, support your pet with topical Helichrysum, Myrrh, Copaiba, Ylang Ylang, Frankincense, and Cypress. Diffuse Protective Blend or Frankincense daily.

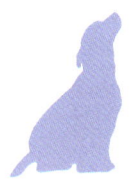

FOR DOGS

Apply 1 drop each Helichrysum, Oregano, Copaiba, Ylang Ylang, Frankincense, and Cypress in 4 tsp. carrier oil twice daily.

Insert a toothpick in the regulator cap of Protective Blend and add this amount of oil to the food 1–2 times daily. On alternate days, insert a toothpick in the regulator cap of Lemon and add this amount of oil to the food 1–2 times daily.

Diffuse Protective Blend or Frankincense at least 20–30 minutes 2–3 times daily.

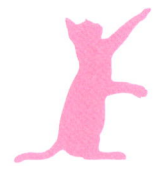

FOR CATS

Apply 1 drop each Helichrysum, Myrrh, Copaiba, Ylang Ylang, Frankincense, and Cypress diluted in 4 tsp. carrier oil twice daily.

Diffuse Protective Blend or Frankincense at least 20–30 minutes 2–3 daily.

Note: Although there are reports of essential oils eliminating heartworms in dogs, we recommend traditional therapies and medications for treatment of this serious illness. In fact, the safest practice is strict control of mosquitoes. We recommend essential oil-based flea, tick and mosquito prevention in conjunction with administration of a monthly heartworm preventative chewable tablet or topical (See Fleas, Ticks and Mosquitoes).

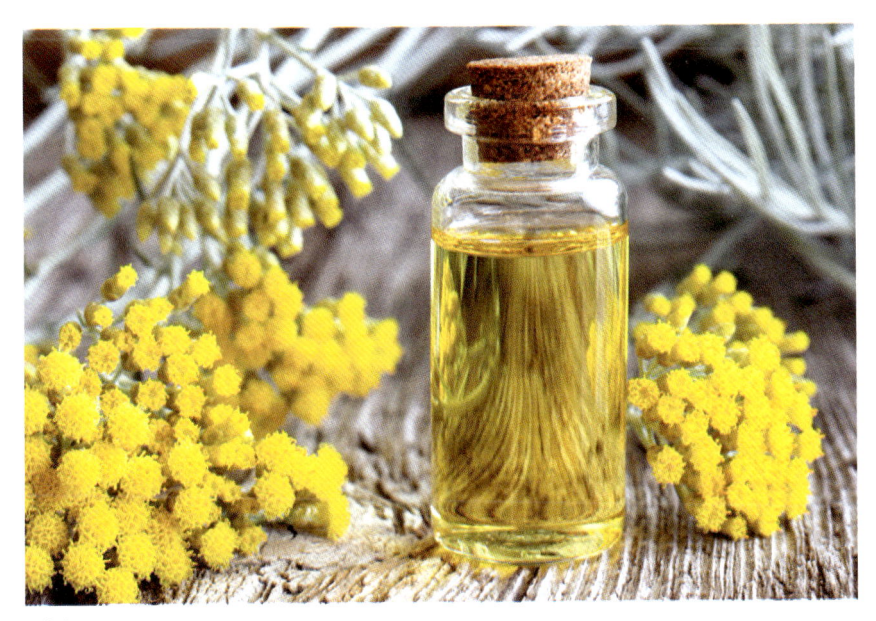

Helichrysum

"No home is complete without the pitter patter of kitty feet."

-Unknown

HEAT STROKE (HYPERTHERMIA)

Pets overheat very easily. For this reason, never leave your pet in the car on a hot or warm day. Pets can suffer heat stroke (Hyperthermia) even if the car windows are open. When spending time outside in the warmer weather, bring water, seek breaks in the shade and watch your pet carefully. It is best to be prepared, so if you are planning an outing in warmer weather, we recommend packing some first-aid oils in case they are needed (See First Aid).

Signs of heat stroke include panting, excessive salivation, pale or red gums, difficulty breathing, disorientation, lack of coordination, passing out or seizures. A pet's normal body temperature is between 100–102.5 degrees Fahrenheit. The most accurate method of taking a pet's temperature is rectally.

Heat stroke is an emergency. Seek Veterinary Care Immediately. This condition requires monitoring in the hospital and intravenous fluid therapy. Many pets suffering from hyperthermia are in shock, so do not waste time offering your pet water. They generally will not drink water in this condition.

When a pet's body temperature becomes too high, brain damage or even death may ensue. Quickly reduce your pet's body temperature by applying cold water compresses to the paws and abdomen. For dogs, apply Peppermint, Massage Blend or Respiratory Blend to the inside of the ear flaps, paws, abdomen and inner thighs. Be cautious when applying oils to your dog's ears as to ensure that no essential oil gets into the eyes (this pertains to dogs with long, floppy ears). Administer Peppermint diluted in a carrier oil safe for ingestion by applying the diluted peppermint to your finger tip and rubbing onto your dog's gums. For cats, apply Massage Blend and Lavender topically. For both dogs and cats, apply Frankincense, Helichrysum and Lavender topically 3–4 times daily.

Ailments, Conditions, and Other Issues

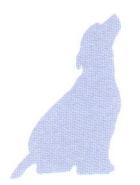

FOR DOGS

Seek veterinary care immediately.

Immediately apply 1 drop Peppermint, Massage Blend or Respiratory Blend diluted in 1 tsp. carrier oil or a pre-diluted roll-on bottle to the ear flaps, paws, abdomen and inner thighs hourly (avoid the eyes) until the dog's body temperature returns to normal. Be cautious when applying oils to your dog's ears as to ensure that no essential oil gets into the eyes (this pertains to dogs with long, floppy ears).

Apply 1 drop each Frankincense, Helichrysum, and Lavender diluted in 1 tsp. carrier oil 3–4 times daily.

Administer 1 drop Peppermint diluted in 1 tsp. of a carrier oil, safe for ingestion, by applying the diluted peppermint to your finger tip and rubbing onto your dog's gums. Monitor your dog's temperature every 15 minutes and repeat if necessary.

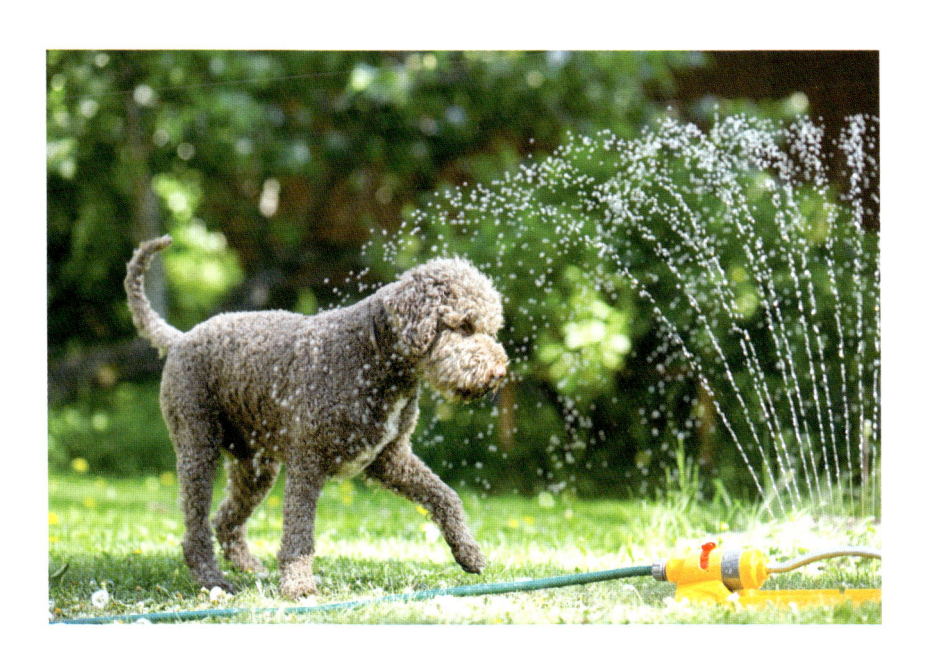

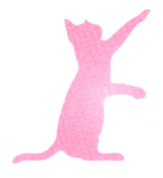

FOR CATS

Seek veterinary care immediately.

Immediately apply 1 drop each Massage Blend and Lavender in 2 tsp. carrier oil to the ear flaps, paws, abdomen and inner thighs hourly (avoid the eyes) until the cat's body temperature returns to normal. Avoid Peppermint in cats.

Apply 1 drop each Frankincense, Helichrysum, and Lavender in 2 tsp. carrier oil 3–4 times daily.

"The world would be a nicer place if everyone had the ability to love as unconditionally as a dog."

-M.K. Clinton

HYPERTHYROIDISM (OVERACTIVE THYROID)

Hyperthyroidism is a common condition in older cats in which the thyroid gland, located in the neck, produces excessive thyroid hormone. Thyroid hormone is crucial to overall health as it affects metabolism, temperature regulation, mood and various other body systems. Cats with hyperthyroidism have too much circulating thyroid hormone which results in an increased metabolism. Basically, the cat's body is in overdrive. Common signs include weight loss despite a ravenous appetite, increased thirst and poor hair coat (See Grooming and Basic Pet Care). Many hyperthyroid cats also develop heart murmurs, heart disease and kidney disease secondarily (See Organ Support). If you notice any of these changes in your cat, consult your veterinarian. Hyperthyroidism requires lifelong support, and cats who take thyroid medication demonstrate a reversal in symptoms. They are less likely to develop complications such as heart disease and kidney disease.

Your veterinarian can diagnose hyperthyroidism with a blood test. Traditional medications are often used to rebalance the amount of thyroid hormone. In addition, support your cat's thyroid gland with essential oils. Apply a combination of Copaiba, Myrrh, Frankincense, and Geranium daily. Diffuse a combination of two of the following: Grounding Blend, Lavender, Geranium, Frankincense, Juniper Berry or Copaiba. Add Grounding Blend and Lavender to the litter box as described in Litter Box Power. In some cases, essential oils may reduce or eliminate the need for medication.

As in all cases, feed your cat a high quality diet supplemented with Omega-3 and probiotics.

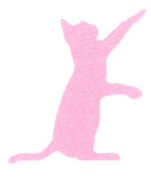

FOR CATS

Apply 1 drop each Copaiba, Myrrh, Frankincense, and Geranium diluted in 4 tsp. carrier oil twice daily.

Diffuse Grounding Blend and Lavender for 20–30 minutes 2–3 times daily.

Add Grounding Blend and Lavender to the litter box as described in Litter Box Power.

Feed your pet a high quality diet supplemented with Omega-3 and probiotics.

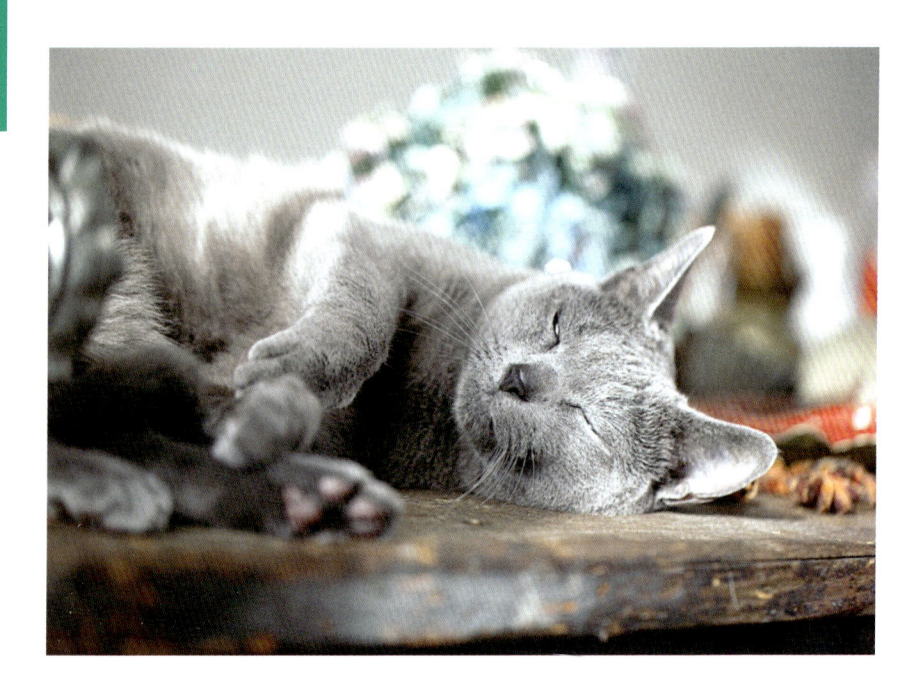

HYPOGLYCEMIA (LOW BLOOD SUGAR)

Young dogs and cats, small puppies and kittens are at the highest risk for hypoglycemia. Most commonly, hypoglycemic puppies and kittens are not eating well, are ill, or are consuming a poor quality food. Young dogs of certain breeds born with a congenital liver shunt may demonstrate signs of hypoglycemia. Other metabolic conditions can decrease blood sugar in pets of all ages (See Organ Support). Another common cause of hypoglycemia is xylitol toxicity. Xylitol is a sweetener found in many household products such as gum, vitamins, medications, antacids and toothpaste. In pets with Diabetes, an overdose of insulin or insulin given without a meal may result in low blood sugar (See Diabetes).

Signs of hypoglycemia include seizures, weakness, collapse, lethargy, disorientation, incoordination and excessive thirst and hunger.

Be careful giving young pets sugar supplements with the intention of maintaining normal blood sugar. These products, which may be falsely marketed as vitamin supplements, often contain primarily high fructose corn syrup, which is taken into the body quickly and results in an immediate rise in blood sugar followed by a rapid decline in blood sugar. Owners are then likely to administer the sugary supplement again, entering a cycle of high and low fluctuations in blood sugar. Rather than sugar supplements, feed a high quality diet several times daily.

If you suspect hypoglycemia, offer your pet food and call your veterinarian. If your pet is too listless to eat, you may offer a liquid sugar product such as Karo syrup via syringe or rub honey or maple syrup on the gums. For dogs and cats, apply Frankincense and Rose. Diffuse Restful Blend or Grounding Blend to reduce stress. See your veterinarian right away.

SpOil Your Pet

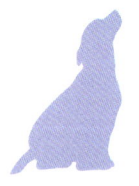

FOR DOGS

Seek veterinary care immediately.

Apply 1 drop each Frankincense and Rose diluted in 2 tsp. carrier oil or a pre-diluted roll-on bottle hourly until your dog is feeling better.

Offer an oral sugar solution.

Diffuse Restful Blend or Grounding Blend for 20–30 minutes 2–3 times daily.

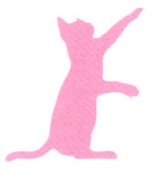

FOR CATS

Seek veterinary care immediately.

Apply 1 drop each Frankincense and Rose diluted in 4 tsp. carrier oil or a pre-diluted roll-on bottle hourly until your cat is feeling better.

Offer an oral sugar solution.

Diffuse Restful Blend or Grounding Blend for 20–30 minutes 2–3 times daily.

HYPOTHYROIDISM (UNDER-ACTIVE THYROID)

Hypothyroidism is a slowed metabolism due to underproduction of thyroid hormone. This condition generally affects middle aged dogs, and certain breeds are more likely to develop an underactive thyroid. Hypothyroidism is very rare in cats. Most of the cases of hypothyroidism are immune-mediated or idiopathic, meaning that no known cause has been identified (See Autoimmune Disorders). In some cases, it is suspected that Hypothyroidism may be associated with environmental toxins, for example household cleaners and air fresheners (See Green Cleaning).

Since thyroid hormone is involved in so many body systems, the signs of hypothyroidism can vary. Most dogs that are affected are lethargic, gain weight and have dry, flaky skin (See Dry Skin). Additional signs include chronic skin and ear infections (See Ear Infections), increased thirst, attraction to heat, seizures (See Seizures) and aggressive and irritable behavior (See Anxiety and Stress). See your veterinarian for a physical exam and appropriate diagnostic testing. Traditionally, hypothyroidism is treated by administering synthetic thyroid hormone.

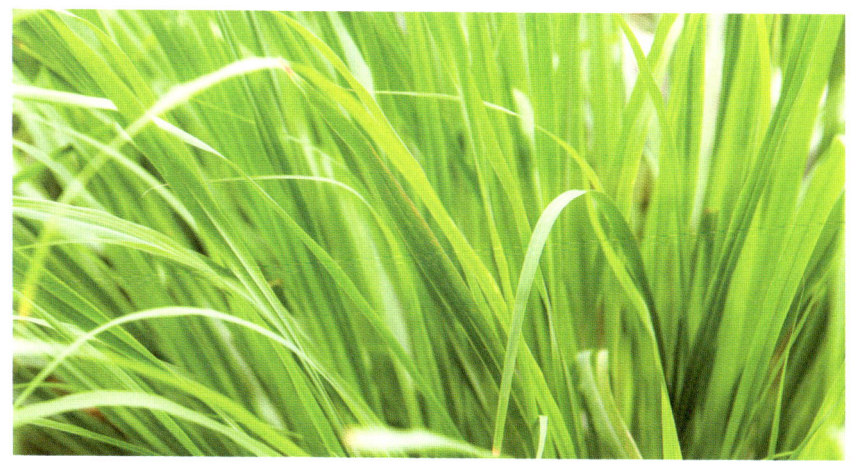

Lemongrass

Essential oils may be used in hypothyroidism to complement traditional therapy and may reduce the amount of medication needed. Apply Lemongrass, Frankincense and Myrrh daily. Diffuse Lemongrass, Frankincense and Myrrh, alternating oils. Add Protective Blend or Lemon to food to support the immune system.

Different essential oils may be used to address your dog's specific symptoms and emotions. Apply or diffuse Joyful Blend, Inspiring Blend or Encouraging Blend to reduce lethargy and depression and increase overall energy. Apply or diffuse Grounding Blend to lessen anxiety and irritability and promote calmness and stability.

Since an underactive thyroid is a chronic condition, which will need to be managed for the rest of your pet's life, consistency of application of essential oils is very important. Always feed your pet a high quality diet supplemented with Omega-3 and probiotics.

"The greatest pleasure of a dog is that you may make a fool of yourself with him, and not only will he not scold you, but he will make a fool of himself, too."

-Samuel Butler

Ailments, Conditions, and Other Issues

FOR DOGS

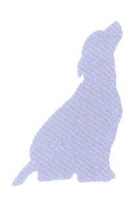

Apply 1 drop each Lemongrass, Frankincense, and Myrrh in 1 tsp. carrier oil twice daily.

Insert a toothpick in the regulator cap of Protective Blend and add this amount of oil to the food 1–2 times daily. On alternate days, insert a toothpick in the regulator cap of Lemon and add this amount of oil to the food 1–2 times daily

For Thyroid Health: Diffuse Lemongrass, Frankincense and Myrrh for 20–30 minutes 2–3 times daily, alternating oils.

For Energy: Diffuse either Joyful Blend, Inspiring Blend or Encouraging Blend for 20–30 minutes 2–3 times daily.

For Calming: Diffuse Grounding Blend for 20–30 minutes 2–3 times daily.

Feed your pet a high quality diet supplemented with Omega-3 and probiotics.

Clean and launder with natural cleaners. Use essential oils to purify and create a soothing home environment. Avoid plastic food bowls and toys.

LIPOMAS (FATTY TUMORS)

Lipomas are very common in dogs of all ages and breeds. In some cases, these benign tumors greatly increase in size, becoming not only unsightly, but may also interfere with the pet's ability to walk, run or play comfortably. Any lump, bump or growth should be evaluated by your veterinarian.

Essential oils are helpful to reduce the size of a lipoma/fatty tumor, thereby reducing your pet's discomfort and increasing mobility. Applying essential oils when a lipoma/fatty tumor is first noticed, may prevent it from increasing in size and interfering with your pet's healthy activity. In addition, essential oils may deter your pet from licking or biting the lipoma/fatty tumor.

Massage the lipoma with Lime or Grapefruit and Frankincense and Copaiba which have beed found to be anti-tumoral. Consistent application will offer the best outcome. Results may take several months.

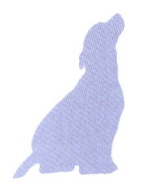

FOR DOGS

A diagnosis from your veterinarian is recommended.

Massage the lipoma with 1 drop Lime or Grapefruit, and 1 drop each Frankincense and Copaiba diluted in 1 tsp. carrier oil 2–4 times daily.

Consistent application will offer the best outcome. Results may take several months.

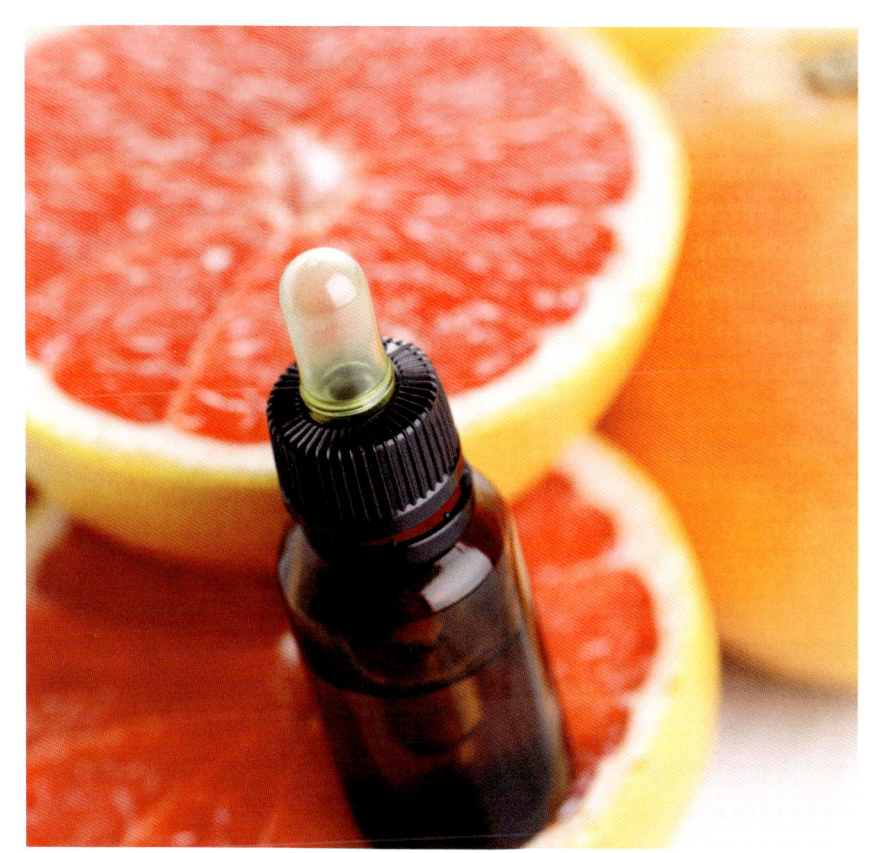

Grapefruit

"Cats are the natural companions of intellectuals. They are silent watchers of dreams, inspiration and patient research."

- Dr. Fernand Mery

LITTER BOX POWER

Many cats and kittens are difficult to medicate, especially once they are aware of their owners' intent, no matter how benevolent it may be. One technique to influence our cats' behavior or to treat illness is to add an essential oil(s) to the litter box. To do this, add 2–3 drops of the chosen essential oil to 1 cup of baking soda. Allow the mixture to rest overnight in a glass jar. Add 1 tablespoon of the mixture of essential oil and baking soda recipe to the litter box daily. The aromatic benefits of the essential oils will be released into the air as your cat steps in the box and paws at the litter. We recommend providing a second litter box which does not contain essential oils to allow the cats time to acclimate to the new litter box. Once you are sure that your cat is not experiencing any adverse effects, you may remove the untreated litter box or add the essential oil mixture to all litter boxes in the home.

Essential oils added to the litter box may help alleviate a number of conditions. For example, add Digestive Blend for cats who suffer from inflammatory bowel disease, vomiting, diarrhea or stress colitis. A nervous or anxious cat may benefit from Lavender added to the litter box, especially in a busy home, filled with visitors or when you go away on vacation. Choose Cleansing Blend, Lemongrass, or Rosemary to control odors naturally.

There are many benefits to using essential oils in the litter box. As mentioned, the primary benefit is to help to maintain health and wellness for your cat. In addition, the use of chemically scented litter has been found to be associated with a number of diseases and illnesses. We strongly suggest that you avoid fragrances and use natural litter box products.

Litter Box Power

Ingredients
2–3 drops Essentail Oils
1 Cup Baking Soda
Glass Jar or Plastic Container*

Instructions
Add 2–3 drops of the chosen essential oil(s) to 1 cup of baking soda. Allow the mixture to rest overnight in a glass jar. Add 1 Tbsp. of the mixture of essential oil and baking soda recipe to the litter box daily.

Some of Our Favorite Combinations

For Calming: Add 1 drop each Lavender, Copaiba and Roman Chamomile Essential Oils

For Digestive Issues: Add 1 drop each Digestive Blend, Myrrh and Lavender Essential Oils

For Kidney and Bladder Issues: Add 1 drop each Juniper Berry and Ylang Ylang or Lavender Essential Oils

For Overall Health: Add 1 drop each Frankincense, Copaiba, and Lavender Essential Oils

For Odor Control: Add 2 drops Cleansing Blend or Rosemary Essential Oils

For Pain: Add 1 drop each Lavender, Frankincense, and Copaiba Essential Oils

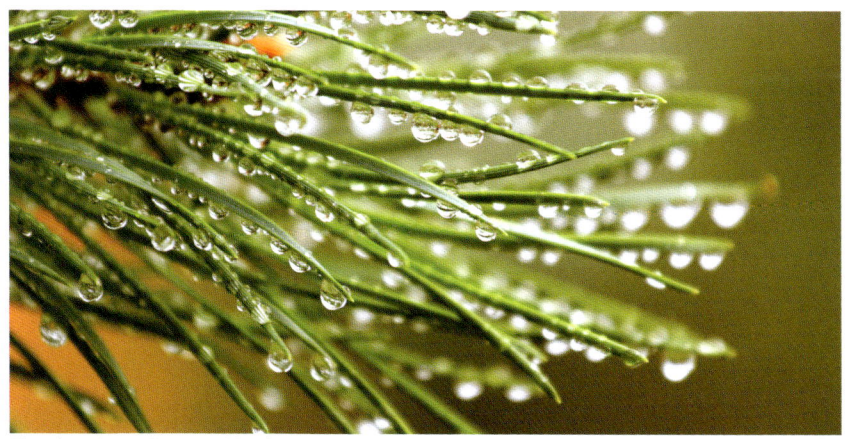

Pine, found in a cleansing blend

LONGEVITY: A LONG AND HEALTHY LIFE

We love our pets! They are family members, and they deserve only the best. We strive to give our pets the longest, healthiest life possible. Optimize your pet's health by using powerful, therapeutic, safe and gentle essential oils.

Pets of any age, from a very your puppy or kitten to elderly, can benefit from the support of essential oils. Caring for a very young puppy or kitten and caring for an older animal is the same, as their systems are sensitive and more susceptible to illness.

It is important that we our knowledgable about the possible health issues that might be associated with individual breeds. Certain breeds are prone to specific health issues and diseases. Being proactive and using an essential oil such as Frankincense, offers overall support and an enhanced and improved quality of life.

- Frankincense is considered the "life force" essential oil. It is very safe for all ages from newborn to elderly. In this book, you'll notice that Frankincense is mentioned in numerous sections and for a variety of conditions.
- Frankincense is one of the oils that crosses the blood-brain barrier, making it useful in neurologic conditions, emotional balance, depression, and in supporting the immune system.
- Frankincense increases oxygen delivery to cells, aiding in respiratory conditions and normal blood pressure levels.
- Frankincense repairs DNA, assisting in treating cancers and autoimmune disease.
- Frankincense is anti-inflammatory and anti-infectious.
- When in doubt, use Frankincense!
- Apply a few drops of Frankincense to your pet daily. This will help to keep your pet healthy, will help to create a bond between you and your pet and will make your young or old pet feel secure.

Ailments, Conditions, and Other Issues

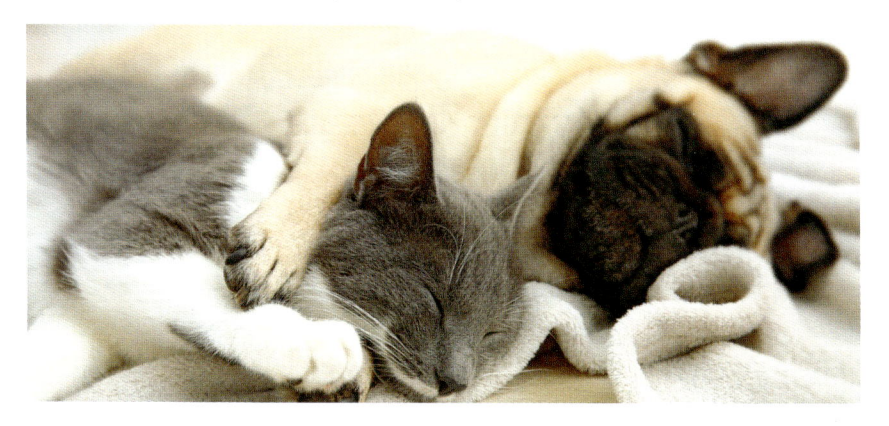

Caring For Your Pet-Young And Old

- Create a comfortable and safe environment for your pet with easy access to food, water, litter box (for cats), and bedding.
- Plenty of regular attention, exercise and affection is good for morale, both yours and your pet's.
- Keep up with routine preventive care such as vaccinations, parasite prevention, dental care and nutritional management.
- Schedule regular wellness exams.
- Monitor your pet and take note of any changes in health or behavior.
- Adjust your pet's nutrition with development and age.
- Make sure your home is at a comfortable temperature.
- Be aware of specific issues relevant to your pet's age and breed.

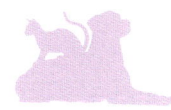

FOR DOGS & CATS

Apply 1 drop Frankincense in 1 tsp. carrier oil for dogs or 2 tsp. carrier oil for cats; or use a pre-diluted roll-on to your pet twice daily

LUMPS AND BUMPS (CYSTS, PAPILLOMAS, WARTS)

As you pet, bathe or brush your pet, have you felt any lumps or bumps on their body? Unsightly growths are very common in pets, especially as pets age. Many lumps, bumps, skin tags and cysts develop randomly, yet some, such as papillomas and warts are often caused by viruses. Cysts are often the result of blocked hair follicles. Certain dog breeds may be more likely to develop skin growths. Pets with a weakened immune system and increased exposure to household cleaners and chemicals may be more at risk (See Green Cleaning). The group of growths discussed in this section is benign and is limited to the skin (See Lipomas, Cancer).

See your veterinarian to evaluate any change in your pet's skin.

Essential oils have been shown to be very effective in treating skin growths, particularly warts and supporting the immune system. In dog breeds that are more susceptible to lumps and bumps, we recommend starting essential oils at a young age. We have found Frankincense, Myrrh, Sandalwood and Lavender to be very valuable.

For warts in dogs, apply Oregano (diluted in dogs), and Arborvitae and Melissa. For cats, apply Melissa, Lavender and Myrrh to the area of concern daily. The wart or growth may appear worse initially, then, fall off. Subsequently, the skin will heal over the next several days. For immune support, diffuse Protective Blend daily. For other benign growths, essential oils may prevent the growth from increasing in size and may even reduce its size. Apply Frankincense, Myrrh, and Lavender on all lumps, bumps and growths daily. To promote healing and immune support always feed your pet a high quality diet and supplement with Omega-3 and probiotics.

Ailments, Conditions, and Other Issues

FOR DOGS

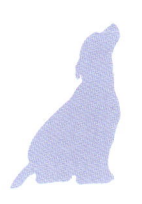

Warts: Apply 1 drop each Oregano, Arborvitae and Melissa in 2 tsp. carrier oil 2–3 times daily.

Diffuse Protective Blend 20–30 minutes 2–3 times daily.

Feed your pet a high quality diet supplement with Omega-3 and probiotics.

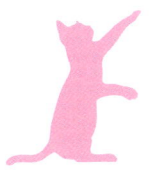

FOR CATS

Warts: Apply 1 drop each Melissa, Lavender and Myrrh diluted in 4 tsp. carrier oil 2–3 times daily.

Diffuse Protective Blend 20–30 minutes 2–3 times daily.

Feed your pet a high quality diet supplement with Omega-3 and probiotics

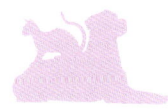

FOR DOGS & CATS

Lumps, Bumps and Growths: Apply 1 drop each Frankincense, Myrrh and Lavender diluted in 1 tsp. for dogs and 2 tsp. for cats 2–3 times daily.

Diffuse Protective Blend 20–30 minutes 2–3 times daily.

Feed your pet a high quality diet supplement with Omega-3 and probiotics.

MASTITIS

Mastitis is inflammation and/or infection of the mammary glands which may develop during nursing of puppies or kittens. The mammary glands become red, inflamed, hard and painful. Milk production may decrease, and the newborns may fail to grow well.

If the mother is feverish, not eating well or refusing to nurse, see your veterinarian. Monitor the puppies' or kittens' growth by weighing them on a gram scale every 2-3 days. If they are not gaining weight, contact your veterinarian.

Clean the mother's mammary glands with Gentle Cleanser 1-2 times daily. Pat dry and apply Healing Salve 2-4 times daily. Try to apply the salve at times of the day when the puppies or kittens are less likely to be nursing, so that the salve may be absorbed well.

For dogs, apply Lavender, Copaiba, Geranium and Myrrh 2-4 times daily. Add Protective Blend to food and give Copaiba by mouth to decrease inflammation and discomfort.

For puppies, apply Frankincense well absorbed to your hands, and pet your puppy, and diffuse Protective Blend to support your new born puppy's immune system. To alleviate any stress in the household, diffuse or apply Lavender or Restful Blend to yourself and the mother twice daily.

For cats, apply Lavender, Copaiba, Geranium and Myrrh twice daily. For kittens, apply Frankincense well absorbed to your hands, and pet your kitten, and diffuse Protective Blend to support your new born kitten's immune system. To alleviate any stress in the household, diffuse or apply Lavender or Restful Blend to yourself and the mother twice daily.

Ailments, Conditions, and Other Issues

FOR DOGS

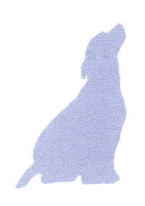

Clean the mother's mammary glands 1–2 times daily with Gentle Cleanser.

Apply 1 drop each Lavender, Copaiba, Geranium and Myrrh diluted in 1 tsp. carrier oil 2–4 times daily.

Apply Healing Salve to the mammary glands 2–4 times daily.

Insert a toothpick in the regulator cap of Protective Blend and add this amount of oil to the food 1–2 times daily.

Administer 1 Copaiba Softgel (for dogs over 30 lbs.) 1–2 times daily. For smaller dogs, insert a toothpick in the regulator cap of Copaiba and add this amount of oil to the food 1–2 times daily.

Diffuse Protective Blend, Restful Blend or Lavender 2–3 times daily.

For puppies, apply 1 drop of Frankincense diluted in 2 tsp. carrier oil daily. Make sure the oil is well absorbed into your hands before application.

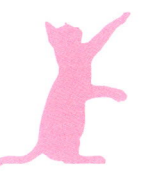

FOR CATS

Apply 1 drop each Lavender, Copaiba, Geranium and Myrrh diluted in 2 tsp. carrier oil 2–4 times daily.

Apply Healing Salve to the mammary glands 2–4 times daily.

Diffuse Protective Blend, Restful Blend or Lavender 2–3 times daily.

For kittens, apply 1 drop of Frankincense diluted in 4 tsp. carrier oil daily. Make sure the oil is well absorbed into your hands before application.

Gentle Cleanser

Ingredients
4 oz. Castile soap or unscented natural foaming soap
2 drops Roman Chamomile Essential Oil
2 drops Lavender Essential Oil
Glass or Plastic Container*

Instructions
Add essential oils to glass or plastic container. Top with soap. Shake the bottle well before use. Lather and rinse well.

Healing Salve

Ingredients
8 oz. Cold-Pressed Organic Coconut Oil
1 oz. Beeswax
2 drops Vitamin E (optional)
10 drops Lavender Essential Oil
5 drops Myrrh Essential Oil
3 drops Helichrysum Essential Oil
Glass Jars , Tin Containers or Plastic Bottle *

Instructions
Place the coconut oil and beeswax over a double –boiler, and gently warm over low heat until the beeswax melts. Remove from heat and add the essential oils and Vitamin E oil, (if using). Quickly pour the mixture into glass jars, tins, or plastic containers and allow to cool completely. Store salve in a cool location where it will not re-melt and re-solidify. When stored correctly, salve will last for 1–3 years. Yields 8 oz.

Ailments, Conditions, and Other Issues

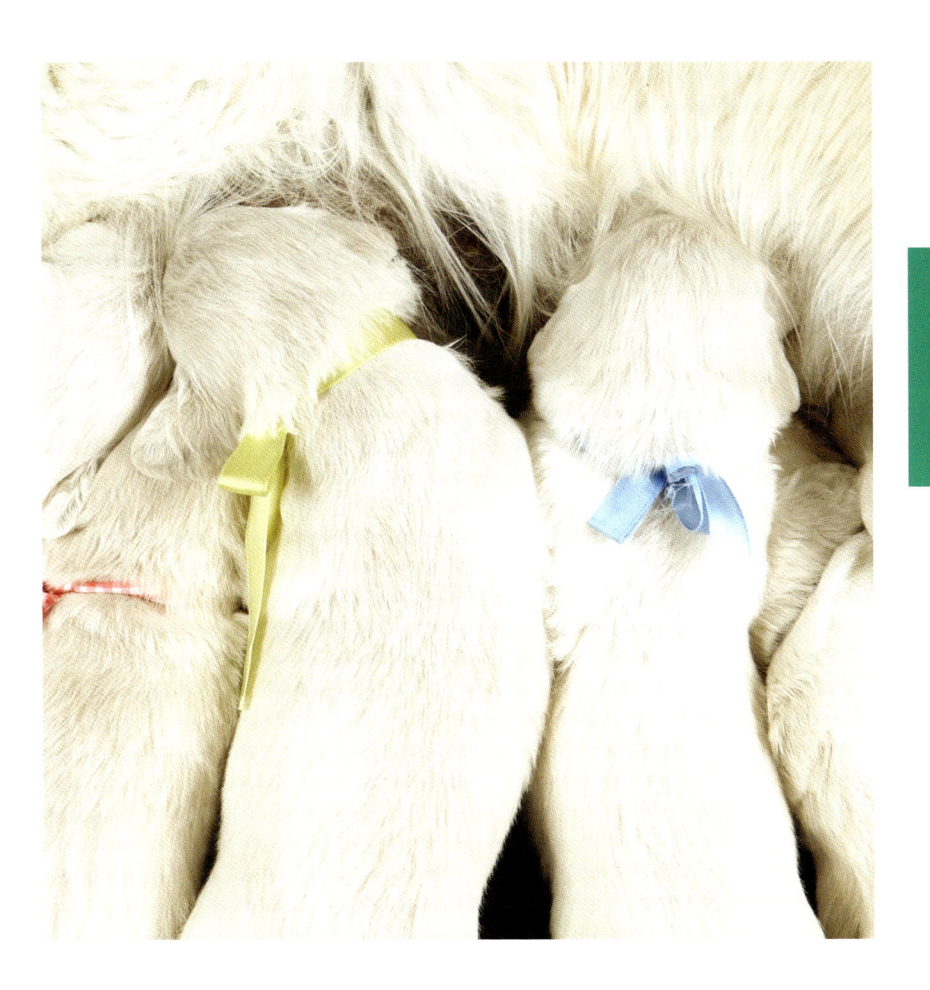

NEW PET PARENTS / INTRODUCING A NEW PET

Congratulations on your new pet! Introducing a new pet into your home with or without other pets is a big change for both you and your pet. Be patient. Many pets take weeks to months to fully acclimate.

Practice close supervision. Confining a new puppy or dog to 1–2 rooms, usually the kitchen, will allow you to watch him or her more carefully. As he or she becomes comfortable, is housebroken and proves to be trustworthy, the allotted space may be increased. When you are not home or not able to provide supervision, we suggest that your new puppy or dog be confined to a crate.
Crate training is a wonderful way to advance your puppy/dog's training, help him/her feel secure, and protect the puppy/dog from causing itself harm or damage. Crates can act as a safety zone, simulating a den, for your dog/puppy. Crates should not be viewed as a punishment nor should be used to punish your puppy/dog.

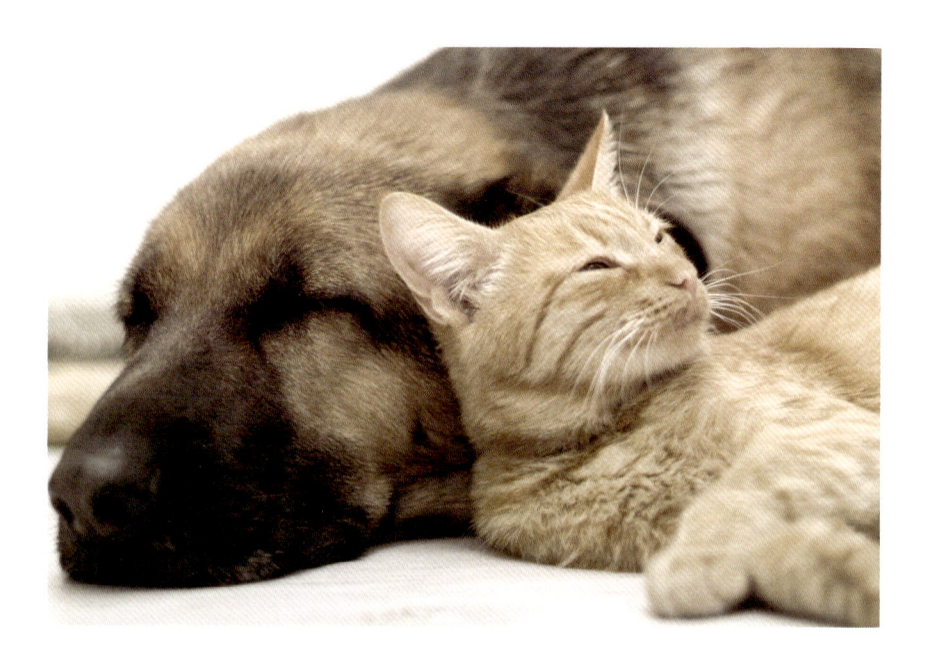

Ailments, Conditions, and Other Issues

Keep a new kitten or cat in one room with food, water, and a litter box. Allow other cats to sniff and paw at him or her under the door. After 1–2 weeks and a thorough veterinary exam, your new addition may explore a greater area of the home while you are present. Be sure the litter box is accessible. The general rule is to provide 1 litter box per cat plus one extra in various locations throughout your home. Scoop the litter boxes daily, and fully clean them weekly (See Recipes: Litter Box Power).

Allow contact or play between pets only under supervision until you feel comfortable that they are amicable. To ease this transition, apply or diffuse a combination of some of the following: Bergamot, Reassuring Blend, Copaiba, Restful Blend and Grounding Blend daily as needed. These oils are especially helpful when you expect moments of agitation, stress, or nervousness. Soft music and dim lighting also promote restfulness and calming. For pets that are nervous or taking a long time to adjust to their new home, apply Frankincense and Juniper Berry twice daily. Juniper Berry is particularly helpful in fearful pets. In ancient cultures, the emotion of fear is concentrated in the kidney area, and Juniper Berry is supportive to the kidneys.

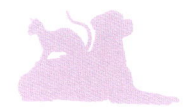

FOR DOGS & CATS

Apply 1 drop each Restful Blend, Copaiba, and Grounding Blend in 1 tsp. for dogs, 2 tsp. for puppies and cats, and 4 tsp. for kittens 2–4 times daily.

For difficult transitions, add 1 drop each Frankincense and Juniper Berry to the above combination.

Diffuse equal parts Restful Blend or Reassuring Blend, Bergamot, Copaiba and Grounding Blend as needed.

NUTRITION—THE FOUNDATION OF HEALTH

Nutrition is the foundation of good health for your pet. A healthy, balanced diet optimizes your pet's immune system, their organ function, and helps them to live long and healthy lives. Good health is built upon a base of excellent nutrition.

Essential oils help deliver nutrients to all the cells of the body. Applying essential oils to your pet or adding essential oils to your dog's food or giving your dog essential oil enhanced supplements is an easy and effective way to increase the availability and absorption of nutrition. For dogs and cats, apply Frankincense daily. For dogs, offer Frankincense and Copaiba internally to support the immune system, nervous system and cellular health and longevity. For cats, apply Lavender and Myrrh. Myrrh stimulates the immune system, aids in blood circulation and promotes tissue regeneration. Two supplements, a probiotic and Omega-3 (fish oil), are especially important, even if your pet eats a high quality diet. A probiotic and a fish oil supplement are not only valuable for excellent general health, they provide benefits particularly helpful for animals affected by seasonal and other allergies. Since most of the immune system resides in the gut, a probiotic directly supports a healthy immune system as well as fortifies the digestive system. Fish oil reduces inflammation in the body, which contributes to a number of diseases. It is beneficial in maintaining healthy skin and a shiny coat.

Feed your pet a high quality diet. Be sure that the first ingredient is a protein such as beef, lamb, fish, chicken or soy and that all of the ingredients are recognizable, compared to a list of unpronounceable chemicals. Beyond these basics, you may look for phrases such as human grade, no by-products, no genetically modified ingredients (GMOs) and organic to indicate the high degree of quality of the pet food. There is research indicating GMOs may negatively impact your pet's health and digestive system. High quality pet foods are sold at stores dedicated to pets or by your veterinarian.

A recent surge of grain-free diets have arrived on the market. Grain-free formulas are ideal for pets with known food allergies, particularly allergies to grains. Grain-free diets do not contain ingredients such as wheat, corn, rice, oats and barley. Some pets with digestive issues, skin sensitivities, or seasonal allergies may also benefit from a grain-free diet. For most other pets, grain-free formulas are optional. Some pets suffer protein allergies and may require a very specific diet (See Allergies).

Some pet foods are fortified with Omega fish oils and probiotics. The benefit of a probiotic is only received if a few criteria are met. The probiotic is a high enough concentration of varied bacterial organisms, can survive stomach acid and digestion and remains viable to establish a stable bacterial population in the intestinal tract. We suggest supplementing your pet's diet with probiotics because the likelihood of pet food meeting these requirements is questionable.

Supplements such as glucosamine and chondroitin sulfate, beneficial for joint health, may also be found in pet foods. For older pets who suffer from arthritis and for pets with other causes of joint pain, the amount of these supplements may not be at a therapeutic dose to bring relief and comfort (See Pain, Arthritis).

An added benefit of a high quality pet food is often evident in the yard or litter box. A highly digestible diet (one without fillers) produces less fecal matter. Although a high quality diet may cost more initially, most pets eat less since every bite is full of good, digestible nutrition. Interestingly, most high quality pet foods are not advertised on television. Choose a pet food that your pet likes, is affordable, and is also convenient for you to find in your local pet store or online.

FOR DOGS

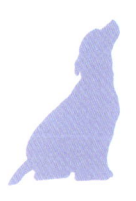

Insert a toothpick in the regulator cap of Frankincense and add this amount of oil to the food 1–2 times daily.

Administer 1 Copaiba Softgel (for dogs over 30 lbs.) 1–2 times daily. For smaller dogs, insert a toothpick in the regulator cap of Copaiba and add this amount of oil to the food 1–2 times daily.

Apply 1 drop Frankincense in 1 tsp. carrier oil twice daily.

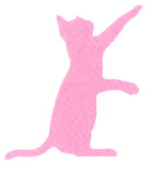

FOR CATS

Apply 1 drop each Frankincense, Lavender and Myrrh diluted in 2 tsp. carrier oil twice daily

OBSESSIVE-COMPULSIVE DISORDER (OCD)

Obsessive-Compulsive Disorder (OCD) can develop for a number of reasons, most commonly, moving to a new home, welcoming a new baby, or changes in family work schedules. Causes of such anxiety may be breed-associated or hereditary, the result of prior maltreatment or abuse, neglect, boredom or nervousness. Obtaining as much history about your pet can be advantageous, but sometimes, the source of stress or anxiety cannot be easily identified. Both dogs and cats can suffer from OCD in different ways (see Anxiety).

Cats with OCD tend to overgroom to the point of removing their hair, termed psychogenic alopecia. Additionally, they may refuse to use the litter box and hide.

Some dogs with this condition tend to lick or bite at their front legs, paws or flanks (the area between the last rib and the rear leg), causing severe wounds and permanent damage to the skin. The skin may be so badly damaged that it scars and may never grow hair back (see Cuts and Scrapes). Other dogs circle repeatedly, chase their tails, chew furniture or other household items, or lick the sofa or bedspread for extended periods of time.

See your veterinarian for a physical exam and appropriate diagnostic testing to rule out any possible medical cause. OCD may be so severe that some pets need traditional medication to prevent them from harming or endangering themselves. Talk to your veterinarian or consult a behaviorist for assistance.

Essential oils offer complementary therapy and may reduce the amount of medication needed and may even eliminate the need for medication.

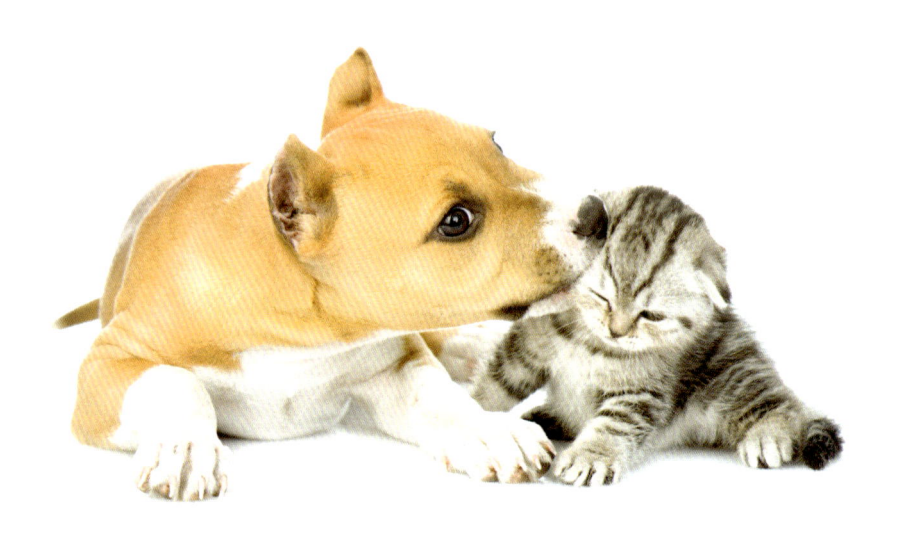

"In order to keep a true perspective of one's importance, everyone should have a dog that will worship him and a cat that will ignore him."

- Derek Bruce

Help calm your pet(s) with Restful Blend and Grounding Blend. Diffuse Calming Blend and Grounding Blend, alternating essential oils. You may find that your pet responds best to a particular oil or to a specific application method, such as using a spray, diffuser, or topical application. For example, a spray vs. direct topical application vs. diffusing. Your pet may also be more anxious during different times of the day or night depending on the activity in the household and may benefit from essential oils during these particular times.

For severe cases of OCD in dogs, try applying a combination of three to four of the following: Frankincense, Cedarwood, Bergamot, Copaiba, Comforting Blend, Reassuring Blend, Restful Blend, Grounding Blend and Women's Perfume Blend daily. For dogs that lick excessively, topical application of Lavender soothes the skin and deters licking.

For cats, apply a combination of two to three of the following: Frankincense, Lavender, Cedarwood, Bergamot, Copaiba, Comforting Blend, Reassuring Blend, Restful Blend, Grounding Blend and Women's Perfume Blend daily. For cats that are overgrooming, topical application of Lavender soothes the skin and deters licking. Add Restful Blend or Grounding Blend to the litter box as described in Litter Box Power.

Lastly, pets are very sensitive to our moods and stress levels. We lead very busy lives and rush around trying to handle our jobs, home, and family life. Use any of the essential oils listed above to help you remain balanced. The calmer you are, the calmer your pets will be.

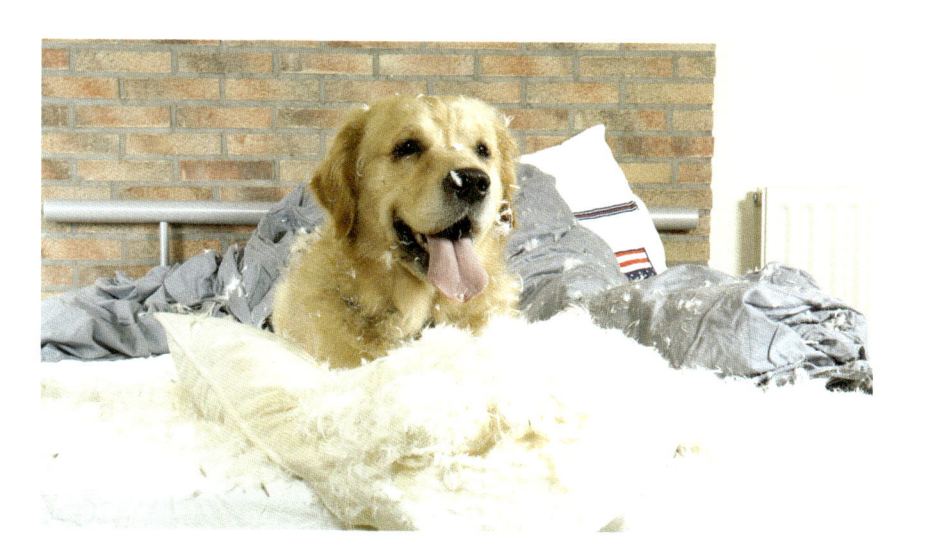

SpOil Your Pet

FOR DOGS

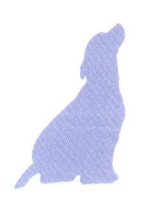

Apply 1 drop each Restful Blend and Grounding Blend diluted in 1 tsp. carrier oil twice daily.

Diffuse Calming Blend and Grounding Blend for at least 20–30 minutes 2–3 times daily .

For severe cases of OCD, combine 5 drops each Frankincense, Lavender, Cedarwood, Copaiba, Restful Blend, Grounding Blend and Women's Perfume Blend in 2 tsp. carrier oil and apply 3–4 times daily. Diffuse Restful Blend and Grounding Blend at least 20–30 minutes 2–3 times daily.

For excessive licking, apply 1 drop Lavender in 1 tsp. carrier oil twice daily or as needed to area of concern.

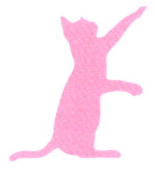

FOR CATS

Apply 1 drop each Restful Blend or Lavender diluted in 1 tsp. carrier oil twice daily.

Diffuse Restful Blend and Grounding Blend at least 20–30 minutes 2–3 times daily.

Add Restful Blend or Grounding Blend to the litter box as described in Litter Box Power.

For severe cases of OCD, combine 1 drop each Frankincense, Lavender, Cedarwood, Copaiba, Restful Blend, Grounding Blend and Women's Perfume Blend in 2 tsp. carrier oil and apply 3–4 times daily.

For overgrooming, apply 1 drop Lavender in 2 tsp. carrier oil twice daily or as needed to area of concern.

Ailments, Conditions, and Other Issues

ORGAN SUPPORT: HEART, KIDNEY & LIVER DISEASE

Heart, Liver and Kidney conditions should be closely monitored by your veterinarian.

Heart disease most often develops as pets age. In some cases, it may be the result of a congenital defect or Heartworm Disease (See Heartworm). As heart disease progresses, the heart enlarges, and puts stress on the circulatory and respiratory systems (See Respiratory Conditions). Most often this will appear as a chronic cough, lethargy, inability to exercise and labored breathing.

Liver disease can develop in pets as they age. In some cases, it may be congenital, the result of infections, toxins, chemicals, and cleaning products (See Green Cleaning). Signs of liver disease, are vomiting, diarrhea, lethargy, and anorexia (See Diarrhea and Vomiting, Anorexia). In more severe cases, your pet may appear jaundiced-a yellowish discoloration to skin, eyes, ears and gums.

Kidney disease is often associated with old age and can also result from infections, metabolic diseases, toxins, chemicals, and cleaning products. Some signs are increased thirst and urinations, and weight loss.

Essential oils may offer organ support and reduce the amount of medications your pet needs. Topical Detoxification Blend supports optimum function by cleansing out toxins from liver, kidneys and bladder, helping these organs to work more efficiently. All pets benefit from good hydration, sleep, proper nutrition, Omega-3 and probiotic supplements to support and strengthen their immune system.

For dogs with Heart Disease (Cardiac Disease), apply Helichrysum, Copaiba and Ylang Ylang daily. To support the respiratory system and easeful breathing, apply and diffuse Respiratory Blend,

Cardamom or Eucalyptus. To improve blood circulation, apply Massage Blend or Cypress and Lavender daily. Diffuse Comforting blend to support your dog emotionally.

For cats with Heart Disease (Cardiac Disease), apply Helichrysum, Copaiba and Ylang Ylang daily and add Helichrysum to the litter box as described in Litter Box Power (See Recipes: Litter Box Power). To support the respiratory system and easeful breathing, apply and diffuse Frankincense or Cardamom. To improve blood circulation, apply Massage Blend or Cypress and Lavender daily. Diffuse Comforting blend to support your cat emotionally.

For dogs with Kidney Disease (Renal Disease and Hypertension), apply Copaiba, Marjoram, Ylang Ylang, Juniper Berry and Helichrysum daily to aid kidney function and give Copaiba orally.

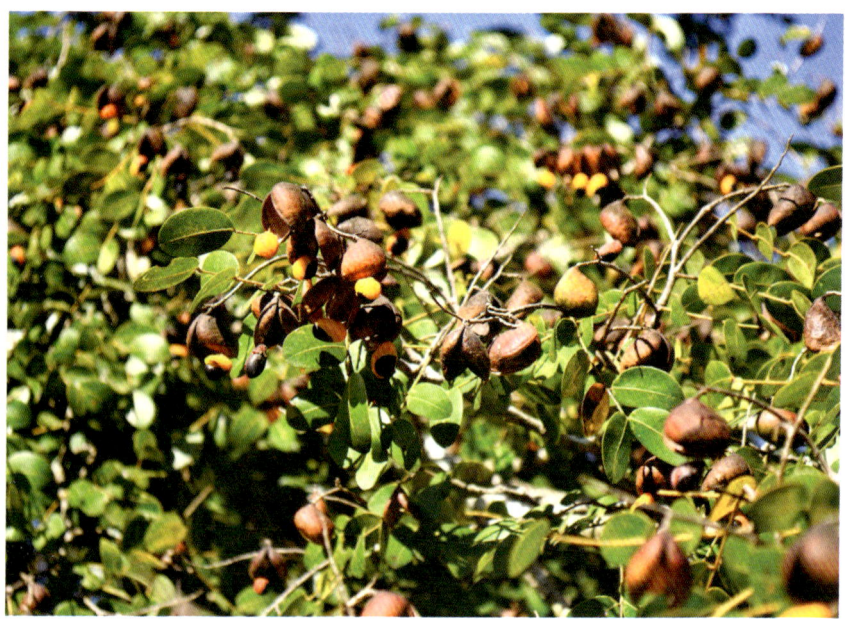

Copaiba

Ailments, Conditions, and Other Issues

These oils will aid in removing toxins in the body and improve hypertension/decrease blood pressure. Diffuse Uplifting Blend and/or Joyful blend to support your dog emotionally. For cats with Kidney Disease (Renal Disease and Hypertension), apply Copaiba, Marjoram, Ylang Ylang, Juniper Berry and Helichrysum daily to aid kidney function and add Juniper Berry and Ylang Ylang or Lavender to the litter box as described in Litter Box Power to help to remove toxins and improve hypertension/decrease blood pressure. Diffuse Uplifting Blend and/or Joyful blend to support your cat emotionally.

For dogs with Liver Disease (Hepatic Disease), apply Rosemary, Geranium, Helichrysum and Myrrh, and/or apply Detoxification Blend which contains many of these oils. Give Copaiba and Detoxification Blend internally. Diffuse Renewing Blend to support your dog emotionally.

For cats with Liver Disease (Hepatic Disease), apply Rosemary, Geranium, Helichrysum and Myrrh daily and/or apply Detoxification Blend which contains many of these oils. Add Geranium and Myrrh to the litter box as described in Litter Box Power. Diffuse Renewing Blend to support your cat emotionally.

SpOil Your Pet

FOR DOGS

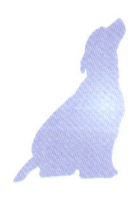

Heart Disease: Apply 1 drop each Helichrysum, Copaiba and Ylang Ylang in 1 tsp. carrier oil twice daily.

Apply 1 drop Respiratory Blend, Cardamom, or Eucalyptus in 1 tsp. carrier oil or a pre-diluted roll-on bottle twice daily.

Apply 1 drop Massage Blend or 1 drop each Cypress and Lavender diluted in 1 tsp. carrier oil 1–2 times daily.

Diffuse Respiratory Blend or Eucalyptus for at least 20–30 minutes 2–3 times daily.

Diffuse Comforting Blend for at least 20–30 minutes 2–3 times daily.

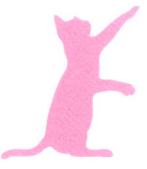

FOR CATS

Heart Disease: Apply 1 drop each Helichrysum, Copaiba and Ylang Ylang in 2 tsp. carrier oil twice daily.

Apply 1 drop Massage Blend or 1 drop each Cypress and Lavender in 2 tsp. carrier oil twice daily.

Apply 1 drop Frankincense or Cardamom diluted 2 tsp. carrier oil twice daily.

Diffuse Frankincense or Cardamom for at least 20 minutes 2–3 times daily.

Diffuse Comforting Blend for at least 20 minutes 2–3 times daily.

Add Helichrysum and Ylang Ylang to the litter box as described in Litter Box Power.

Ailments, Conditions, and Other Issues

FOR DOGS

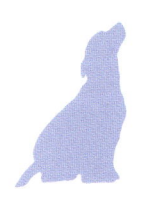

Kidney Disease: Apply 1 drop each of Copaiba, Marjoram, Ylang Ylang, Juniper Berry and Helichrysum diluted 2 tsp. carrier oil twice daily.

Administer 1 Copaiba Softgel (for dogs over 30 lbs.) 1–2 times daily. For smaller dogs, insert a toothpick in the regulator cap of Copaiba and add this amount of oil to the food 1–2 times daily.

Diffuse Uplifting Blend or Joyful Blend for at least 20 minutes 2–3 times daily.

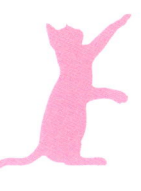

FOR CATS

Kidney Disease: Apply 1 drop each of Copaiba, Marjoram, Ylang Ylang, Juniper Berry and Helichrysum diluted in 4 tsp. carrier oil twice daily.

Add Juniper Berry and Ylang Ylang or Lavender to the litter box as described in Litter Box Power.

Diffuse Uplifting Blend or Joyful Blend for at least 20 minutes 2–3 times daily.

FOR DOGS

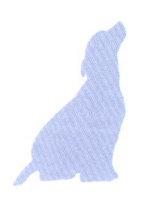

Liver Disease: Apply 1 drop each Rosemary, Geranium, Helichrysum and Myrrh diluted in 2 tsp. carrier oil and/or apply 1 drop Detoxification Blend diluted in 2 tsp. carrier oil twice daily.

Administer 1 Copaiba Softgel (for dogs over 30 lbs.) 1–2 times daily. For smaller dogs, insert a toothpick in the regulator cap of Copaiba and add this amount of oil to the food 1–2 times daily. Administer 1 Detoxification Softgel (for dogs over 70 lbs.). For smaller dogs (between 30–70 lbs.) add 1 drop Detoxification Blend to an empty veggie capsule. For dogs less than 30 lbs., insert a toothpick in the regulator cap of of Detoxification Blend and add this amount of oil to the food 1–2 times daily.

Diffuse Renewing Blend for at least 20 minutes 2–3 times daily.

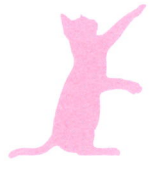

FOR CATS

Liver Disease: Apply 1 drop each Rosemary, Geranium Helichrysum and Myrrh and/or apply 1 drop Detoxification Blend diluted in 4 tsp. carrier oil twice daily.

Add Geranium and Myrrh to the litter box as described in Litter Box Power.

Diffuse Renewing Blend for at least 20 minutes 2–3 times daily.

PAIN

Pain is so powerful that it actually inhibits healing and suppresses the immune system. Signs of pain include vocalization, restlessness or agitation, abnormal posture, difficulty moving around, trembling, reduced appetite, licking or biting. You may also notice a faster than normal heartbeat and rapid breathing.

For dogs, apply Massage Blend, Helichrysum, Lavender, Marjoram, Myrrh, Tumeric or Copaiba. A polyphenol supplement containing extracts from Frankincense Gum Resin, Curcumin (Turmeric), Ginger Root, Green Tea, Pomegranate Fruit, Grape Seed, and Resveratrol and an oral preparation of Copaiba offer powerful relief from soreness and discomfort (See Arthritis).

For cats, apply Massage Blend, Helichrysum, Lavender, Marjoram, Turmeric or Myrrh. Add Lavender, Frankincense and Copaiba to the litter box as described in Litter Box Power.

"They motivate us to play, be affectionate, seek adventure, and be loyal."

–Tom Hayden

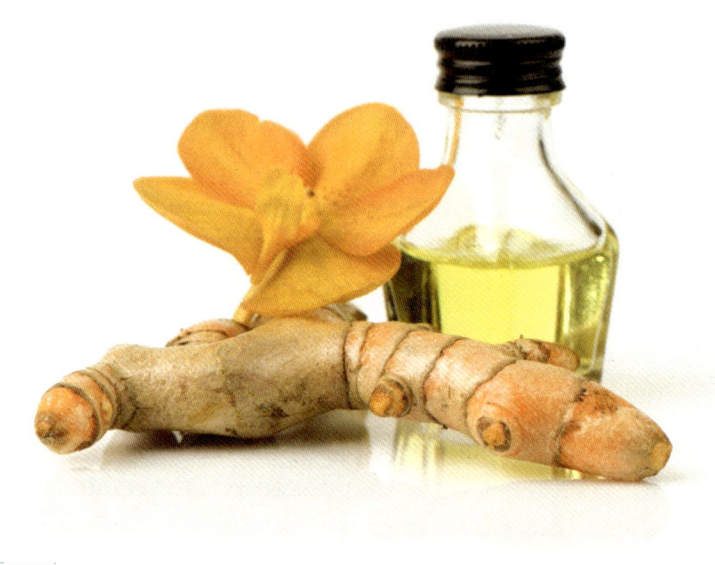

Turmeric

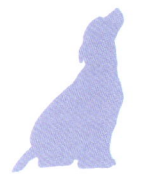

FOR DOGS

Apply 1 drop each Massage Blend, Marjoram, Copaiba, Turmeric and any ONE of the following oils: Helichrysum, Myrrh or Lavender diluted in 2 tsp. carrier oil 2–4 times daily.

Administer 1 Polyphenol Complex (for dogs over 45 lbs.) and/or 1 Copaiba Softgel (for dogs over 30 lbs.) 1–2 times daily. For smaller dogs, insert a toothpick in the regulator cap of Copaiba and add this amount of oil to the food 1–2 times daily.

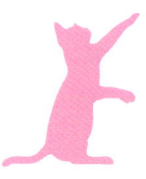

FOR CATS

Dilute 1 drop each Massage Blend, Myrrh, Copaiba and ONE of the following oils: Helichrysum, or Lavender in 4 tsp. carrier oil 1–2 times daily.

Add Lavender, Frankincense, and Copaiba to the litter box as described in Litter Box Power.

PANCREATITIS

Pancreatitis is a very painful condition in which the pancreas becomes inflamed. Pets with pancreatitis are ill. Signs include vomiting (more common in dogs), anorexia, lethargy, depression and weight loss (especially in cats). Due to a painful abdomen, pets often have difficulty getting into a comfortable position, are reluctant to lie down and guard their abdomens. Dogs may display "praying position" where their elbows are resting on the floor and their tail area is held up in the air. This position eases abdominal pressure and pain.

Pancreatitis is diagnosed by a physical exam, blood tests, x-rays and ultrasound. Pancreatitis is serious and requires hospitalization, intravenous (IV) fluids, and close medical attention. Call your veterinarian if your pet is showing any of the above signs.

Causes of pancreatitis include overeating, eating foods high in fat, abrupt changes in diet, viruses, and unknown causes. Especially in pancreatitis, it is crucial to feed your pet a high quality diet supplemented with Omega-3 and probiotics. Certain breeds of dogs are predisposed to developing pancreatitis. For those pets prone to pancreatitis, we recommend avoiding table food, high fat treats and snacks and using supportive essential oils like Frankincense and Digestive Blend to protect your pet.

Essential oils can be used to relieve abdominal discomfort, decrease inflammation, and offer your pet symptom relief. Apply Digestive Blend, Frankincense, Lavender, and Massage Blend daily. Administer an oral preparation of Copaiba which offers powerful relief from discomfort and reduce inflammation (See Pain). For cats add Digestive Blend, Frankincense, and Lavender to the litter box (See Recipes: Litter Box Power).

SpOil Your Pet

Diffuse Protective Blend to support your pet's immune system and Restful Blend or Lavender to keep you and your pet calm.

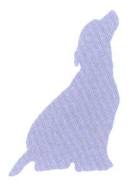

FOR DOGS

Apply 1 drop each Digestive Blend, Frankincense, Copaiba and Massage Blend in 2 tsp. carrier oil 2–4 times daily.

Administer 1 Copaiba Softgel (for dogs over 30 lbs.) 1–2 times daily. For smaller dogs, insert a toothpick in the regulator cap of Copaiba and add this amount of oil to the food 1–2 times daily.

Diffuse Protective Blend for 20–30 minutes 2–3 times daily.

Diffuse Restful Blend or Lavender for 20–30 minutes 2–3 times daily.

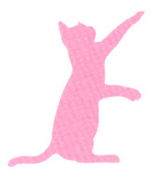

FOR CATS

Apply 1 drop Digestive Blend, Frankincense, Copaiba and Massage Blend in 4 tsp. carrier oil 2–4 times daily.

Add Digestive Blend, Frankincense, and Lavender to the litter box (See Recipes: Litter Box Power).

Diffuse Protective Blend for 20–30 minutes 2–3 times daily.

Diffuse Restful Blend or Lavender for 20–30 minutes 2–3 times daily.

Ailments, Conditions, and Other Issues

POISONING

Pets are often curious. Be sure to keep chemicals, tobacco, alcohol, cleaning products, plants, flowers, medications and vitamin supplements away from pets. (See Burns for a complete list of safety recommendations and for information on chemical burns.)

The two most common chemical toxicities are ingestion of rat poison and antifreeze. Ingestion of antifreeze (ethylene glycol) has the highest fatality rate of all pet poisonings. These products, and all toxic substances, should not be kept anywhere in your home, basement or garage. In addition, certain foods such as chocolate, grapes and raisins are harmful and should be avoided. Xylitol, a common sweetener found in toothpaste, chewing gum, candies and mints is poisonous to dogs and cats. Household and garden plants and flowers such as Lilies, Daffodils, Tulips and Poinsettias, just to name a few, are highly toxic to our pets if ingested. Common over the counter medications, such as acetaminophen and aspirin are highly dangerous. Never administer medication to your pet without consulting your veterinarian.

Signs of poisoning include lethargy, salivation, vomiting, diarrhea, tremors, and seizures.

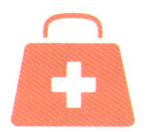

Poisonings are emergencies. Contact Animal Poison Control* and your veterinarian immediately. Always keep contact information for your veterinarian, emergency hospital and animal poison control center handy.

Animal Poison Control Hotline : 1-800-548-2423

Animal Poison Helpline: 1-800-213-6680

SpOil Your Pet

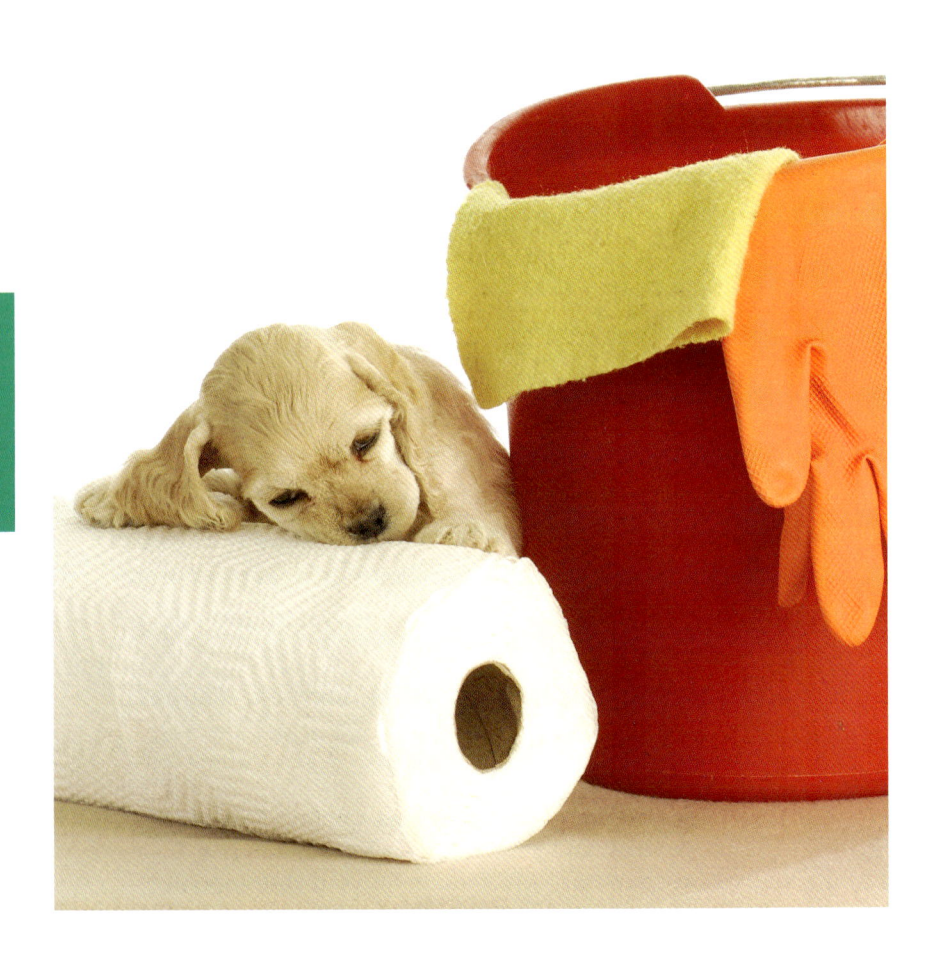

"The gift which I am sending you is called a dog and is in fact the most precious and valuable possesion of mankind."

- *Theodorus Gaza*

Ailments, Conditions, and Other Issues

PRE AND POST-OPERATIVE CARE

During your pet's life he or she may require planned or emergency surgery. No matter whether the surgery is scheduled or not, this can be a very stressful time for both you and your pet. In addition to the stress, keeping your pet healthy prior to surgery is crucial. A strong immune system will help your pet to recover and decrease the possibility of infection. Stress has been found to suppress the immune system and the body's ability to heal. Essential oils, are a valuable component and will help you to prepare and support your pet during the peri-operative period.

Begin to expose your pets to essential oils 5 days prior to surgery, if possible. Prior to surgery, we suggest applying Frankincense and Copaiba to support the immune system. Apply Grounding Blend, Restful Blend, or Reassuring Blend to ease anxiety in the home. Diffusing is a non-intrusive and effective way of enveloping your pet with the healing compounds found in pure essential oils. We recommend diffusing oils that cleanse the air of germs such as Protective Blend and Cleansing Blend. To promote a calm environment, diffuse Grounding Blend, Reassuring Blend or Restful Blend. Incorporating a probiotic in your pet's diet will aid in immune support and help to reduce anxiety (See Anxiety and Stress).

The immediate post-operative period, usually the first 72–96 hours after surgery, is an important time for healing and recovery to take place. Pets may feel uncomfortable, confused, and their normal activities or routine may be compromised. This period can also be a time of adjustment in mobility, learning to wear an elizabethan collar, bandage, or cast. Some pets may feel saddened or depressed. For other pets, who have been in pain, surgery may offer relief from tenderness, and the pet may feel energized and rejuvenated. Some pets impress us by recovering so quickly that they are more active than they should be and try to do too much too soon. The goals during the post operative period are to minimize discomfort, support the immune system, reduce infection and inflammation and hasten complete recovery. Continue to support your pet's immune system, attend to pain and infection control in the post-operative period with essential oils for up to two weeks as needed.

After surgery, to decrease the effects of anesthesia, to support the immune system and prevent infection, apply Helichrysum, Geranium, Frankincense, Copaiba, Myrrh, Lavender and Lemongrass to the body (not on the incision). Apply Healing Salve (See Recipes: Healing Salve) to any wound or incision. For pain management, add Massage Blend.

Diffuse Grounding Blend, Restful Blend or Reassuring Blend to calm the emotions and curtail excess energy. For very active pets, we recommend diffusing a combination of Grounding Blend, Restful Blend, Vetiver and Lavender. Such energetic pets may also benefit from an oral supplement of Copaiba which offers powerful antioxidants, neurological support and helps to relieve anxiety and an oral softgel Restful Blend preparation (Restful Blend oil should not be given orally). We recommend diffusing oils that cleanse the air of germs such as Protective Blend and Cleansing Blend. Ginger has been found to help in post-operative pain and nausea in a recent study and may be added to the diffuser recommendations above.

Ailments, Conditions, and Other Issues

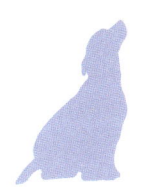

FOR DOGS

5 Days Before Surgery:

Apply 1 drop each Frankincense and Copaiba in 1 tsp. carrier oil twice daily.

Apply 1 drop Grounding Blend, Restful Blend, or Reassuring Blend in 1 tsp. carrier oil twice daily.

Diffuse Protective Blend or Cleansing Blend for 20–30 minutes 2–3 times daily.

Diffuse Grounding Blend, Reassuring Blend or Restful Blend for 20–30 minutes 2–3 times daily.

Feed your pet a high quality diet supplemented with Omega-3 and probiotics.

Post Surgery:

For detoxification of anesthesia: Apply 1 drop each Helichrysum, Geranium, Frankincense, Copaiba, Myrrh, Lavender and Lemongrass in 2 tsp. carrier oil to the body (not on the incision) twice daily for the first 5 days after surgery.

5 - 14 days after surgery: Apply 1 drop each Frankincense, Copaiba, Geranium, Myrrh, and Lavender diluted in 2 tsp. carrier oil twice daily.

Apply Healing Salve to any wound or incision twice daily for 14 days.

For pain: Add 1 drop Massage Blend to the above combination.

Diffuse Protective Blend or Cleansing Blend for 20–30 minutes 2–3 times daily. Ginger may be added to either of these oils for pain management.

Diffuse Grounding Blend, Reassuring Blend or Restful Blend for 20–30 minutes 2–3 times daily. Ginger may be added to one of these oils for pain management.

For very active dogs, we recommend diffusing a combination of 3 drops Grounding Blend, 2 drops Restful Blend, 2 drops Lavender and 1 drop Vetiver in 8 oz./1 cup water for 20–30 minutes 2–3 times daily or more if needed.

SpOil Your Pet

Administer 1 Copaiba Softgel (for dogs over 30 lbs.) 1–2 times daily. For smaller dogs, insert a toothpick in the regulator cap of Copaiba and add this amount of oil to the food 1–2 times daily. Administer 1 Restful Blend Softgel (for dogs over 15 lbs.) 1–2 times daily (Restful Blend oil should not be given orally).

Feed your pet a high quality diet supplemented with Omega-3 and probiotics.

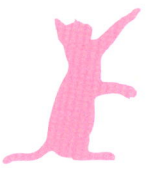

FOR CATS

Post Surgery:

For detoxification of anesthesia: Apply 1 drop each Helichrysum, Geranium, Frankincense, Copaiba, Myrrh, Lavender and Lemongrass in 4 tsp. carrier oil to the body (not on the incision) twice daily for the first 5 days after surgery.

5 - 14 days after surgery: Apply 1 drop each Frankincense, Copaiba, Geranium, Myrrh, and Lavender diluted in 4 tsp. carrier oil twice daily.

Apply Healing Salve to any wound or incision twice daily for 14 days.

For pain: Add 1 drop Massage Blend to the above combination.

Diffuse Protective Blend or Cleansing Blend for 20–30 minutes 2–3 times daily. Ginger may be added to either of these oils for pain management.

Diffuse Grounding Blend, Reassuring Blend or Restful Blend for 20–30 minutes 2–3 times daily. Ginger may be added to one of these oils for pain management.

For very active cats, we recommend diffusing a combination of 3 drops Grounding Blend, 2 drops Restful Blend, 2 drops Lavender and 1 drop Vetiver in 8 oz./1 cup water for 20–30 minutes 2–3 times daily or more if needed.

Ailments, Conditions, and Other Issues

Add Myrrh, Frankincense and Lavender to the litter box as described in Litter Box Power.

Feed your pet a high quality diet supplemented with Omega-3 and probiotics.

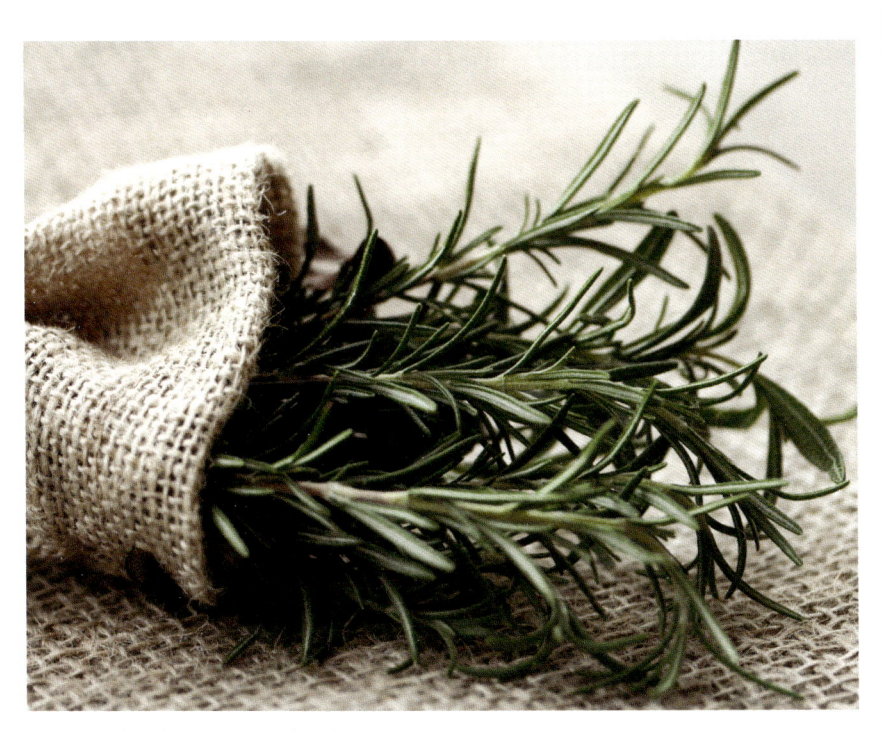

Rosemary, found in a protective blend

PREGNANCY, LABOR AND DELIVERY

Is your pet expecting? How exciting! Keeping the mother healthy during this time is critical so your pet will have an easy pregnancy and delivery and will give birth to healthy new kittens and puppies.

Good nutrition will keep your pet healthy and support your pet during pregnancy and nursing. Feed the mother a high quality puppy or kitten diet, and speak to your veterinarian about additional supplementation. The extra fats, protein and calcium, found in a puppy or kitten diet offer the mother the extra required nutrition needed during pregnancy and lactation.

"Happiness is a warm puppy."

- Charles M Schulz

Essential oils are beneficial for supporting your pet's immune system during pregnancy. Births of any kind are exciting and stressful for all. Essential oils will help to keep you and your pet calm during pregnancy and delivery. Try to prepare a quiet, comfortable area for the mother as the delivery approaches. Essential oils will help ease the stress of an impending birth and create a supportive and healthy environment.

Apply Frankincense and Myrrh to the mother during pregnancy and delivery to prevent infection and to support the immune system. Apply Lavender or Restful Blend throughout the pregnancy, labor and delivery to keep you and the expectant mother calm. Diffuse Frankincense, Roman Chamomile, Restful Blend or Lavender throughout the birthing process to create a calm and healthy atmosphere.

Ailments, Conditions, and Other Issues

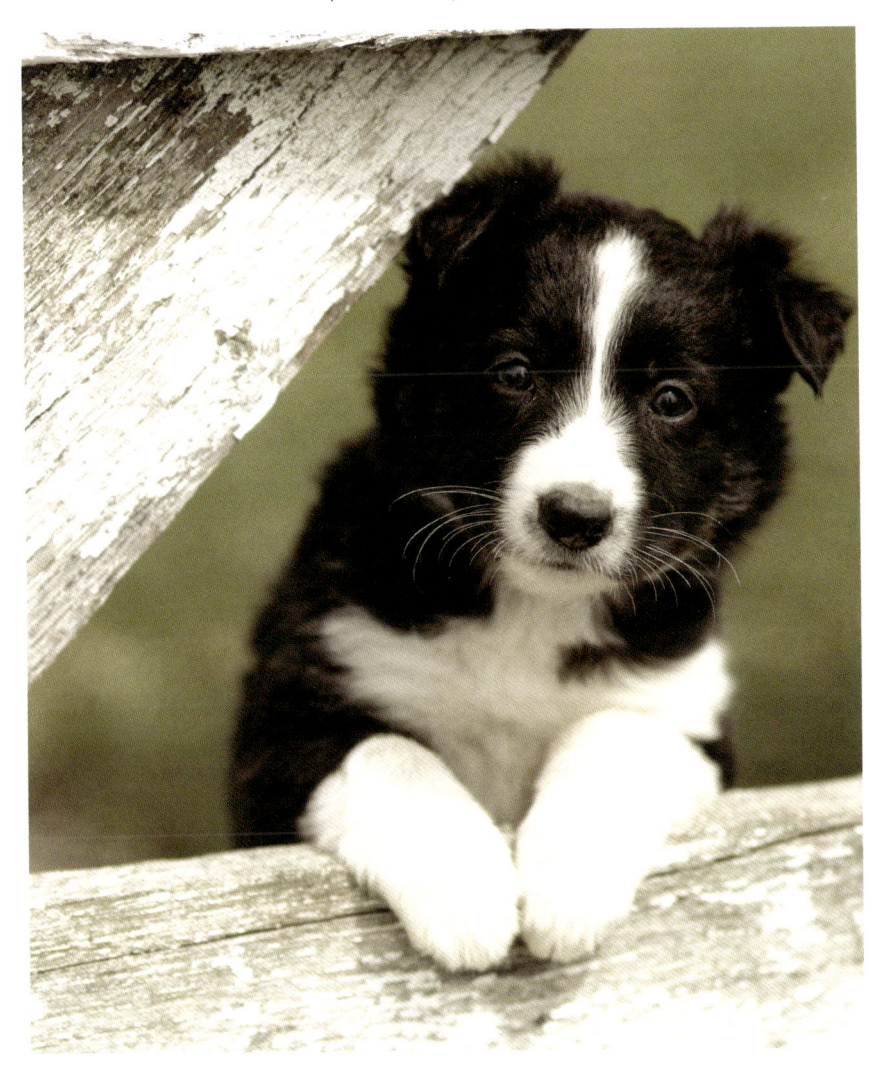

Once the kittens or puppies are born, welcome them into the world with an anointing, on the crown of the head, with Frankincense, and apply Frankincense and Myrrh to the cut umbilical cords.

To foster healthy milk production, lactation, or to increase the mother's milk production, apply Fennel at the onset of labor and during nursing. For dogs, add Fennel to the food.

SpOil Your Pet

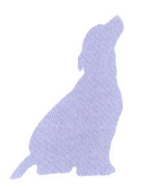

FOR DOGS

Lactation/Nursing: Apply 1 drop Fennel in 1 tsp. carrier oil 2–4 times daily.

Insert a toothpick in the regulator cap of Fennel and add this amount of oil to the food 1–2 times daily.

Feed a high quality puppy food throughout lactation.

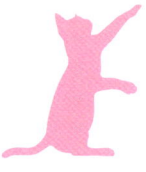

FOR CATS

Lactation/Nursing: Apply 1 drop Fennel in 2 tsp. carrier oil 2–4 times daily.

Feed a high quality kitten food throughout lactation.

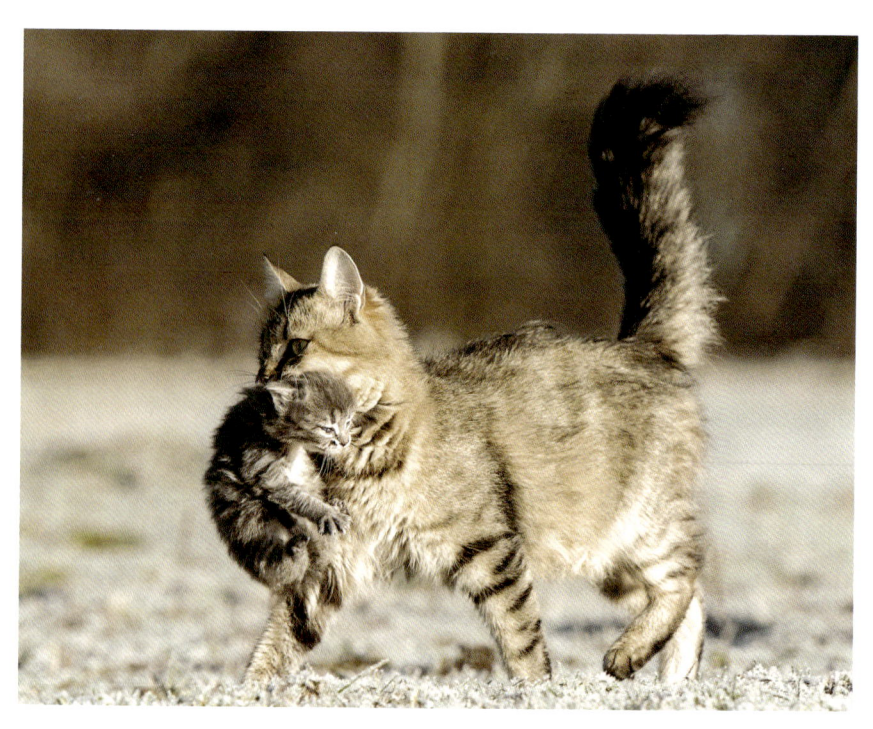

Ailments, Conditions, and Other Issues

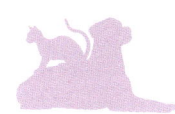

FOR DOGS & CATS

Pregnancy: Apply 1 drop each Frankincense and Myrrh in 1 tsp. carrier oil for dogs and 2 tsp. carrier oil for cats twice daily.

Apply 1 drop each Lavender or Restful Blend in 1 tsp. carrier oil for dogs and 2 tsp. carrier oil for cats twice daily.

Diffuse Frankincense, Roman Chamomile, Restful Blend or Lavender for 20–30 minutes 2–3 times daily.

Feed a high quality puppy or kitten food throughout the pregnancy.

Labor and Delivery: Apply 1 drop each Frankincense and Myrrh in 1 tsp. carrier oil for dogs and 2 tsp. carrier oil for cats every 2 hours.

Apply 1 drop each Lavender or Restful Blend in 1 tsp. carrier oil for dogs and 2 tsp. carrier oil for cats every 2 hours.

Diffuse Frankincense, Roman Chamomile, Restful Blend or Lavender for 20–30 minutes 2–3 times daily.

After Birth: Apply 1 drop Frankincense in 4 tsp. carrier oil to the crown of the head of the newborn.

Apply 1 drop each Frankincense and Myrrh in 4 tsp. carrier oil to the newborns' cut umbilical cords.

Apply 1 drop each of Frankincense and Myrrh in 1 tsp. carrier oil for dogs and 2 tsp. carrier oil for cats to the mother twice daily.

Apply 1 drop Lavender or Restful Blend in 1 tsp. carrier oil for dogs and 2 tsp. carrier oil for cats twice daily to the mother.

Diffuse Frankincense, Roman Chamomile, Calming Blend or Lavender for 20–30 minutes 2–3 times daily.

PROSTATIC DISEASE

Prostatic disease typically affects older male intact (not neutered) dogs, at an average age of 8–9 years. Cats rarely develop prostatic disease. Enlargement of the prostate is directly influenced by testosterone, so neutered males are not affected.

The prostate gland is located at the base of the bladder. If the prostate gland becomes enlarged, it constricts the flow of urine through the urethra. The prostate may also become infected, abscessed or develop cysts See Urinary Conditions).

Signs of prostatic disease include difficulty urinating, discolored or bloody urine, and discharge from the penis. Additional signs are lethargy, loss of appetite, abdominal pain, fever, and vomiting.

See your veterinarian if you notice any of the above signs in your dog. Prostatic disease is diagnosed with a physical exam, blood tests, x-rays and ultrasound. Prostatic disease is treated with antibiotics and by neutering your dog.

Essential oils can assist your dog by reducing inflammation and by fighting bacteria. To reduce inflammation, apply Frankincense, Helichrysum, Copaiba and Lavender daily. An oral preparation of Copaiba will help reduce inflammation and support the immune system. For prostatic infections, secondary urinary tract infections and prostatic abscesses, add Thyme daily. For hormone balance, consider applying Ylang Ylang or Clary Sage. Further support your pet by diffusing immune supporting and calming oils such as Frankincense, Lavender and Grounding Blend.

Ailments, Conditions, and Other Issues

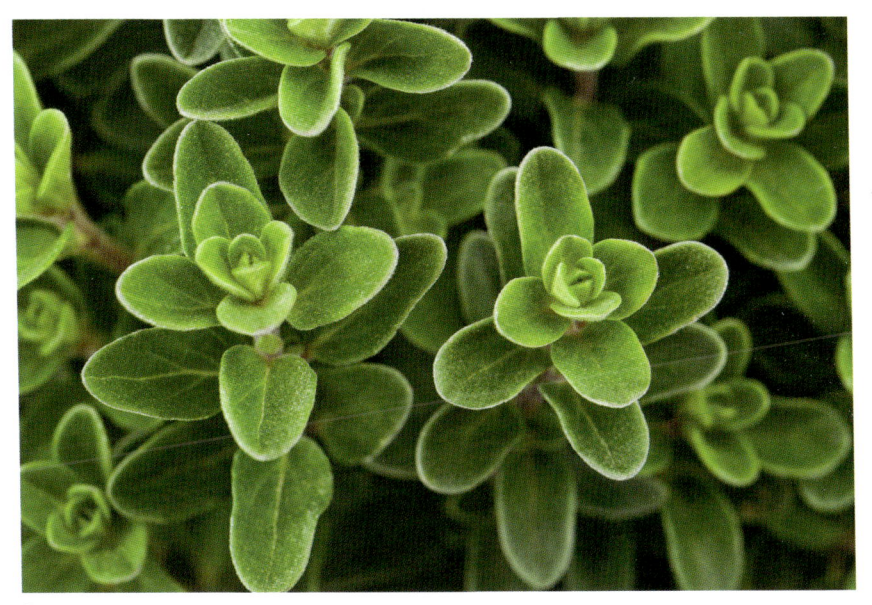

Oregano

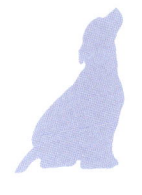

FOR DOGS

Apply 1 drop each Frankincense, Helichrysum, Copaiba and Lavender in 2 tsp. carrier oil twice daily.

Administer 1 Copaiba Softgel (for dogs over 30 lbs.) 1–2 times daily. For smaller dogs, insert a toothpick in the regulator cap of Copaiba and add this amount of oil to the food 1–2 times daily.

For prostatic infections, secondary urinary tract infections and prostatic abscesses, apply 1 drop Thyme in 2 tsp. carrier oil twice daily.

For hormone balance, apply 1 drop Ylang Ylang or Clary Sage in 1 tsp. carrier oil twice daily.

Diffuse Frankincense, Lavender or Grounding Blend for 20–30 minutes 2–3 times daily.

Continue to feed your pet a healthy diet, and supplement with Omega-3 and probiotics.

SpOil Your Pet

PYOMETRA (UTERINE INFECTION)

Pyometra develops in intact (not spayed) female dogs and cats when the uterus becomes infected and fills with pus. Pyometra usually occurs 2 months after a female dog's heat cycle (estrus). Female cats can develop a pyometra at any time in their reproductive cycles. Signs of a pyometra include lethargy, decreased appetite, drinking excessively, fever and, in some cases, vaginal discharge. If the cervix is closed at the time a pyometra develops, the pus is trapped within the uterus and cannot escape. In this situation, vaginal discharge will not be observed, your pet's symptoms may be more pronounced, and your pet may be at greater risk of uterine rupture. If the cervix is open, the pus may drain and be observed externally. Either situation is extremely serious.

If you notice any of these signs, call your veterinarian. A pyometra is an emergency and can be fatal.

Your veterinarian will diagnose a pyometra with a physical exam, blood tests, x-rays and ultrasound. The uterus, quickly filling with pus, is at risk of rupture and must be removed right away. The treatment for a pyometra is to spay your dog or cat immediately. Pets with pyometra often remain in the veterinary hospital and are treated with antibiotics, fluid therapy, and pain relief.

Essential oils can support your pet's immune system, promote healing and fight bacteria. For dogs, apply a combination of Frankincense, Helichrysum, Copaiba and Geranium daily to reduce inflammation. Use a mixture of Thyme, Myrrh, and Lavender daily to limit infection and promote healing. Administer an oral preparation of Copaiba to support the immune system and offer powerful relief from soreness and discomfort. Diffuse Protective Blend for added immune support. Apply Massage Blend as needed for pain (See Pain).

For cats, apply a combination of Frankincense, Helichrysum, Copaiba and Geranium daily. Fight infection and promote healing by applying Thyme, Myrrh and Lavender daily. Daily use of Massage Blend may be used to reduce pain and diffuse Protective Blend to support the immune system.

Ailments, Conditions, and Other Issues

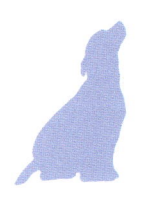

FOR DOGS

Apply 1 drop each Frankincense, Helichrysum, Copaiba and Geranium in 1 tsp. carrier oil 2–3 times daily.

Apply 1 drop each Thyme, Myrrh and and Lavender in 2 tsp. carrier oil 2–3 times daily.

Apply 1 drop Massage Blend in 1 tsp. carrier oil 2–4 times daily as needed for pain.

Administer 1 Copaiba Softgel (for dogs over 30 lbs.) 1–2 times daily. For smaller dogs, insert a toothpick in the regulator cap of Copaiba and add this amount of oil to the food 1–2 times daily.

Diffuse Protective Blend for at least 20–30 minutes 2–3 times daily.

Feed your pet a high quality diet and continue supplementing with Omega-3 and probiotics.

Note: Pyometra is preventable by spaying your dog at a young age, ideally prior to any heat (estrus) cycles.

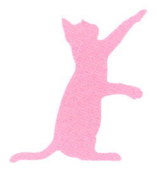

FOR CATS

Apply 1 drop each Frankincense, Helichrysum, Copaiba and Geranium in 2 tsp. carrier oil 2–3 times daily.

Apply 1 drop each Thyme, Myrrh and and Lavender in 4 tsp. carrier oil 2–3 times daily.

Apply 1 drop Massage Blend in 2 tsp. carrier oil 2–4 times daily as needed for pain.

Diffuse Protective Blend for at least 20–30 minutes 2–3 times daily.

Feed your pet a high quality diet and continue supplementing with Omega-3 and probiotics.

Note: Pyometra is preventable by spaying your cat at a young age, ideally prior to any heat (estrus) cycles.

RESPIRATORY CONDITIONS

Respiratory conditions, such as Canine Cough Complex, Feline Asthma, and Kennel Cough, can be the result of several conditions including viruses, bacteria, fungal organisms, parasites, allergies, heart disease and cancer. Dogs and cats are also affected by second-hand smoke (See Second Hand Smoke). Most commonly, pets cough, sneeze, wheeze, and suffer from runny eyes and noses. Some pets cough so much that they vomit (See Diarrhea and Vomiting).

Since signs of respiratory illness can indicate many different issues, it is best to see your veterinarian for a physical exam, diagnostic testing and an appropriate treatment plan which may include essential oils.

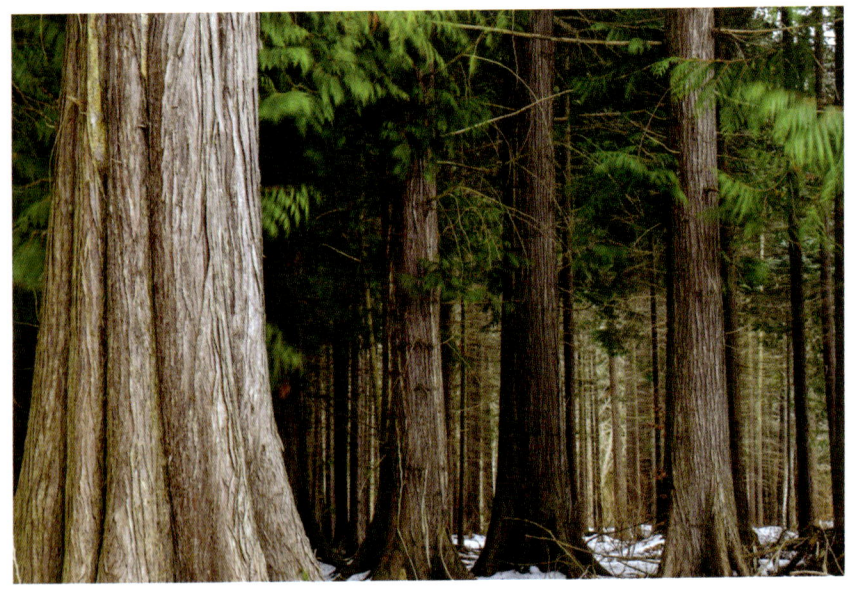

Arborvitae forest

Essential oils are a beneficial adjunct therapy to support your pet. To help your pet breathe more easily and open up airway passages, apply Respiratory Blend and Frankincense topically. Diffuse Protective Blend, Respiratory Blend, or Cleansing Blend for several hours each day and night, especially in the area where your pet

Ailments, Conditions, and Other Issues

sleeps. These will help support the immune system, decrease airborn allergens and germs.

Trouble breathing can be very stressful for you and your pet. Apply and diffuse Restful Blend, Renewing Blend or Lavender to help keep you and your pet calm. Lavender is also anti-viral and a natural antihistamine which is beneficial if your pet is suffering from a virus or allergies.

> *"If you think dogs can't count, try putting three dog biscuits in your pocket and then give him only two of them."*
>
> *- Phil Pastoret*

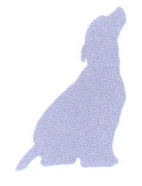

FOR DOGS

Apply 1 drop each Respiratory Blend, Frankincense and Lavender diluted in 2 tsp. carrier oil 2–4 times daily.

Diffuse Protective Blend, Respiratory Blend, Frankincense or Cleansing Blend for several hours each day and throughout the night, especially in the pet's sleeping area.

For Calming: Apply 1 drop of either Restful Blend or Renewing Blend in 1 tsp. carrier oil 2–4 times daily.

Diffuse Restful Blend or Renewing Blend for 20–30 minutes 2–3 times daily.

Continue to support your pet's immune system with a high quality diet, Omega-3 and probiotics.

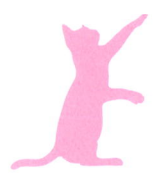

FOR CATS

Apply 1 drop each of Respiratory Blend, Frankincense and Lavender diluted in 4 tsp. carrier oil twice daily.

Diffuse Protective Blend, Respiratory Blend, Frankincense, or Cleansing Blend for several hours each day and throughout the night, especially in the pet's sleeping area.

For Calming: Apply 1 drop of either Restful Blend or Renewing Blend in 1 tsp. carrier oil 2–4 times daily.

Diffuse Restful Blend or Renewing Blend for 20–30 minutes 2–3 times daily.

Continue to support your pet's immune system with a high quality diet, Omega-3 and probiotics.

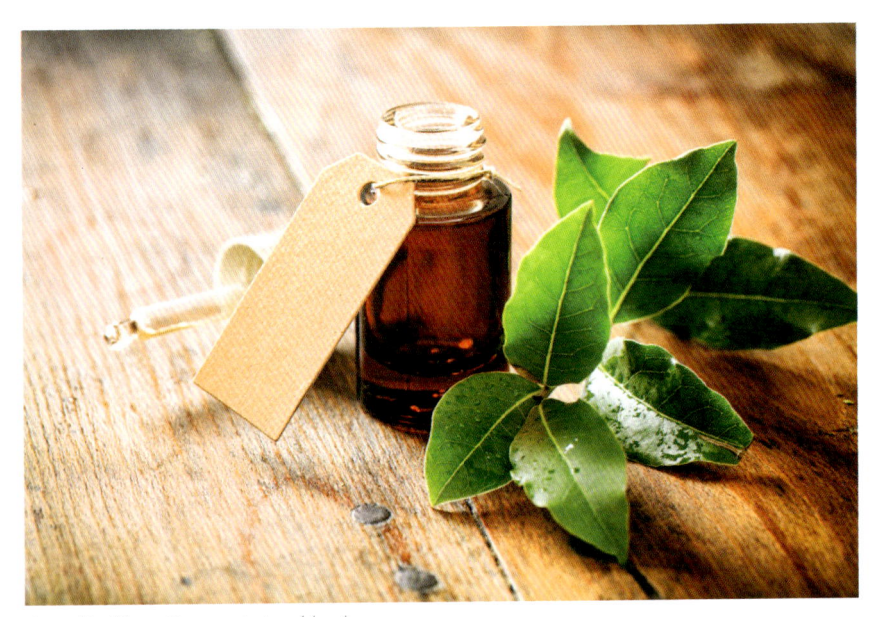

Laurel leaf found in a respiratory blend

Ailments, Conditions, and Other Issues

RINGWORM

Ringworm is a fungal infection, not a worm. Ringworm affects dogs and cats of all ages, but is most common among kittens. It is highly contagious between cats and dogs and may be spread to people. Signs of Ringworm include hair loss, crusty lesions, and scratching. Lesions tend to be found on the ears, face, and front paws. A diagnosis by your veterinarian is recommended. Ringworm is a persistent infection and the treatment may take several weeks to months to cure.

Essential oils are highly effective against fungal infections and help to heal skin lesions. The combination of Geranium, Myrrh, Lemongrass and Lavender have been shown to kill fungal organisms and help to restore and repair skin eruptions. Bathe once to twice weekly using natural essential oil Antiseptic Shampoo. Use caution to avoid the eyes. Since many cats are resistant to bathing, apply Healing Salve, which contains Myrrh and Lavender, to affected areas twice daily. Ringworm infections can be stubborn, and oral antifungal medication may be required. To minimize spread of this infection, launder any washcloths, rags, or towels used to bathe your pet with Protective Blend Laundry Detergent. Keep these contaminated items separate from any other laundry. Diffusing essential oils such as Protective Blend, Frankincense and Lavender will help to support the immune system and reduce stress and discomfort.

Ringworm is highly contagious. Wear gloves while treating or bathing your pet.

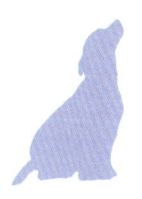

FOR DOGS

Combine 1 drop each Geranium, Myrrh, Lemongrass and Lavender in 2 tsp. carrier oil twice daily. Apply mixture to affected areas, using caution to avoid the eyes.

Bathe once to twice weekly using natural essential oil Antiseptic Shampoo. Use caution to avoid the eyes. Launder any washcloths, rags, or towels used to bathe your pet with Protective Blend Laundry Detergent. Keep these contaminated items separate from any other laundry.

Apply Healing Salve to affected areas twice daily.

Diffuse Protective Blend or Frankincense and Lavender for 20–30 minutes 2–3 times daily.

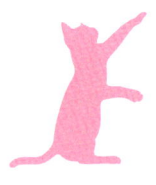

FOR CATS

Combine 1 drop each Geranium, Myrrh, Lemongrass and Lavender in 4 tsp. carrier oil twice daily. Apply mixture to affected areas, using caution to avoid the eyes.

Bathe once to twice weekly using natural essential oil Antiseptic Shampoo. Use caution to avoid the eyes. Launder any washcloths, rags, or towels used to bathe your pet with Protective Blend Laundry Detergent.

Apply Healing Salve to affected areas twice daily.

Diffuse Protective Blend or Frankincense and Lavender for 20–30 minutes 2–3 times daily.

Since many cats are resistant to bathing, oral antifungal medication may be required to reduce or eliminate the need to bathe your cat.

Antiseptic Shampoo

Ingredients
110 oz. Water
2 oz. Aloe Vera
1 Tbsp. Castile soap
2 drops Myrrh Essential Oil
2 drops Lavender Essential Oil
2 drops Geranium Essential Oil
2 drops Cleansing Essential Oil Blend
Glass or Plastic Bottle

Instructions
Add essential oils to an empty bottle. Add castile soap, aloe vera juice and water. Shake the bottle well before use. Lather and rinse well.

Healing Salve

Ingredients
8 ounces Cold-Pressed Organic Coconut Oil
1 ounce Beeswax
2 drops Vitamin E (optional)
10 drops Lavender Essential Oil
5 drops Myrrh Essential Oil
3 drops Helichrysum Essential Oil
Glass Jars or Tin Containers

Instructions
Place the coconut oil and beeswax over a double –boiler, and gently warm over low heat until the beeswax melts. Remove from heat and add the essential oils and Vitamin E oil, (if using). Quickly pour the mixture into glass jars or tins, and allow to cool completely. Store salve in a cool location where it will not re-melt and re-solidify. When stored correctly, salve will last for 1–3 years. Yields 8 oz.

SCABIES (SARCOPTIC MANGE)

Scabies is a highly contagious mite which burrows just beneath the surface of the the skin of dogs. Scabies can infect your dog all year round and effects dogs of all ages and breeds. It is usually spread from dog to dog. The presence of the Sarcoptes scabiei mite causes intense itching. The dog will chew and scratch its skin constantly, resulting in the loss of hair concentrated on the legs and belly. Overtime, this chronic inflammation and irritation causes the skin to become darker and thicker, and secondary bacterial infections are common. If your dog develops skin eruptions, hair loss, or is severely scratching, see your veterinarian. Scabies is diagnosed with a physical exam and microscopic examination of skin scrapings. Traditional treatment includes oral medication, bathing and antibiotics. Since scabies is very contagious, keep your dog away from other dogs, avoid dog parks, doggie day care, boarding and grooming. Scabies can easily infect people, however scabies can not survive in people, so the mites will die in a few days, and the infection is short lived. However, it causes intense itching during that time, and medical treatment is suggested.

Complement traditional therapy with essential oils. Essential oils can soothe the skin, reduce itching, support the immune system and prevent infection. Apply Lavender, Arborvitae, Cleansing Blend, Myrrh and Helichrysum to the affected areas by petting. Apply Healing Salve and/or Sunburn/Skin Healing spray to lesions to heal skin irritation(s) and reduce itching. Bathing your dog using the Antiseptic Shampoo with 3 drops Cleansing Blend added will help keep the skin clean, heal any skin infections and help to remove flaky skin. To minimize spread of this infection, launder any washcloths, rags, or towels used to bathe your pet with Protective Blend Laundry Detergent. Keep these contaminated items separate from any other laundry. Administer an oral preparation of Copaiba to support the immune system and reduce inflammation. Diffusing essential oils such as Protective Blend, Frankincense and

Lavender will help to support the immune system and reduce stress and discomfort.

Feed your pet a high quality diet, and supplement with Omega-3 and probiotics.

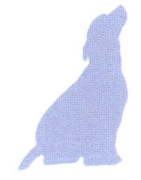

FOR DOGS

Scabies is highly contagious. Wear gloves while treating or bathing your pet.

Apply 1 drop each of Lavender, Arborvitae, Cleansing Blend, Myrrh and Helichrysum in 2 tsp. carrier oil twice daily to affected areas or by petting.

Apply Healing Salve 1–2 times daily to localized lesions.

Apply Sunburn/Skin Healing Spray 2–4 times daily or as needed.

Bathe with Antiseptic Shampoo with 3 drops added Cleansing Blend 1–2 times weekly. Use caution to avoid the eyes. Launder any washcloths, rags, or towels used to bathe your pet with Protective Blend Laundry Detergent.

Administer 1 Copaiba Softgel (for dogs over 30 lbs.) 1–2 times daily. For smaller dogs, insert a toothpick in the regulator cap of Copaiba and add this amount of oil to the food 1–2 times daily.

Diffuse Protective Blend or Frankincense and Lavender for 20–30 minutes 2–3 times daily.

Feed a high quality diet and supplement with Omega-3 and probiotics.

Healing Salve

Ingredients
8 ounces Cold-Pressed Organic Coconut Oil
1 ounce Beeswax
2 drops Vitamin E (optional)
10 drops Lavender Essential Oil
5 drops Myrrh Essential Oil
3 drops Helichrysum Essential Oil
Glass Jars or Tin Containers

Instructions
Place the coconut oil and beeswax over a double –boiler, and gently warm over low heat until the beeswax melts. Remove from heat and add the essential oils and Vitamin E oil, (if using). Quickly pour the mixture into glass jars or tins, and allow to cool completely. Store salve in a cool location where they will not re-melt and re-solidify. When stored correctly, salve will last for 1–3 years. Yields 8 ounces.

Antiseptic Shampoo

Ingredients
10 oz. water
2 oz. Aloe Vera Juice
1 Tbsp. of Castile soap
2 drops of Myrrh Essential Oil
2 drops of Lavender Essential Oil
2 drops of Geranium essential oil
2 drops Cleansing Blend

Instructions
Combine in a jar. Shake well. Lather and rinse well

Sunburn/Skin Healing Spray

Ingredients
4 ounce dark glass spray bottle
1 ounce Aloe Vera Juice
2–4 drops Lavender Essential Oil
1 drop Helichrysum Essential Oil

Instructions
Place all ingredients in the dark glass spray bottle. Shake well. Spray the affected area, taking caution to avoid your pet's eyes. You may spray some of the mixture into your hands and carefully apply to your pet's face, head and muzzle.

Note: Try to purchase the best quality Aloe Vera Juice possible. Aloe Vera products which contain synthetics will dry the skin and will not help the skin to heal from the sunburn or skin condition.

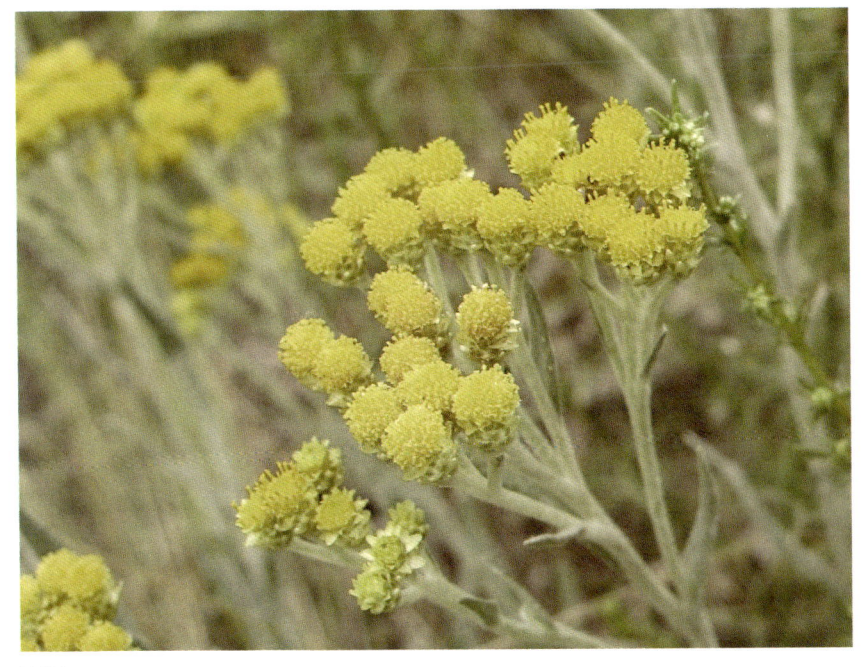

Helichrysum

SEIZURES AND NEUROLOGIC CONDITIONS

A variety of conditions can lead to seizures and neurologic disease in dogs and cats. Seizures are most commonly inherited or due to metabolic diseases, hypoglycemia, trauma, toxins, viral infections, and tumors (See Cancer, Poisoning and Green Cleaning). Seizures occur because of uncontrollable abnormal electrical impulses in the brain. Many of us think of the body shaking violently and convulsing, yet some seizures are much more subtle. Seizures may appear as small muscle twitches of the eyelids, whiskers or ears, whole body trembling or uncontrolled movements of one leg. Other possible signs are repeated and excessive behaviors such as biting or licking at the air and licking of the lips. If you notice any of these signs contact your veterinarian. It may be helpful to record on video and in writing details of such events if opportunity allows.

Neurologic conditions can lead to seizures and are often observed as loss of balance, falling, circling, head tilt, dizziness and abnormal eye movements. These may be the result of hereditary disease, congenital malformations of the brain and spinal column, pain, tick-borne illness, severe or chronic ear infections, vestibular disease and tumors (See Fleas, Ticks and Mosquitoes, Tick-Borne Diseases and Ear Infections).

If your dog or cat is having a seizure, consult your veterinarian. Use caution when applying essential oils while your pet is having a seizure to avoid being injured. In particular, being bitten, scratched or kicked while your pet is unaware of his or her actions. Frankincense, Rose, Jasmine, Copaiba and Helichrysum are especially beneficial and calming to the nervous system. Keeping you and your pet relaxed during a seizure is very important. Several essential oils such as Grounding Blend, Roman Chamomile, Restful Blend, Joyful Blend,and Lavender may be used to reduce tension in the home.

Ailments, Conditions, and Other Issues

Nutrition is crucial to supporting your pet's brain and nervous system. If your pet is prone to seizures, we suggest speaking to your veterinarian about a neuro- protective diet high in medium chain triglycerides (MCTs). Current research shows that coconut oil, high in MCTs, may support the brain and may be helpful in reducing seizures and improving cognitive impairments. In dogs with a breed predisposition to seizures and neurologic disease, we suggest feeding a high quality diet supplemented with coconut oil, Omega-3 and probiotics (See Nutrition).

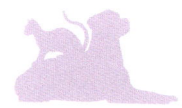

FOR DOGS & CATS

Seek veterinary care immediately.

Be careful applying oils while your pet is having a seizure.

Apply a pre-diluted roll-on of Rose or Jasmine to the palms of your hands. To this, add a combination of 1 drop each Frankincense, Copaiba and Helichrysum and 1 drop each of two of any of the following oils: Grounding Blend, Roman Chamomile, Restful Blend, Joyful Blend or Lavender in 2 tsp. carrier oil for Dogs and 4 tsp. carrier oil for cats twice daily or as needed.

Diffuse Frankincense, Lavender, or Restful Blend for at least 20–30 minutes 2–3 times daily.

SEPARATION ANXIETY

Have you ever had the misfortune of walking into your house to find overturned furniture, inches-deep claw gouges on door frames, blood-stained tooth marks on window sills, and countless messages on your answering machine from neighbors complaining about your dog barking and howling for hours on end in your absence? If so, you're probably familiar with the term "separation anxiety" – a mild label for a devastating and destructive behavior.

Separation anxiety is a condition in which animals exhibit symptoms of anxiety or excessive distress when they are left alone. The most common separation anxiety symptoms in dogs include destructive behavior, house soiling, trembling, pacing, and excessive vocalization. Many dogs with this challenging behavior also refuse to eat or drink when left alone, don't tolerate crating, pant and salivate excessively when distressed, and go to great lengths to try to escape from confinement, with apparent total disregard for injury to themselves or damage to their surroundings.

It's natural for young mammals to experience anxiety when separated from their mothers and siblings; it's an adaptive survival mechanism. A pup who gets separated from his family cries in distress, enabling Mom to easily find him and rescue him. In the wild, even an adult canine who is left alone is more likely to die – either from starvation, since he has no pack to hunt with, or from attack, since he has no pack mates for mutual protection. For this reason, signs of separation anxiety in puppies is somewhat expected. This behavior should not be mistaken for disobedience or spite. Our pets are quite distressed in our absence. Although it is difficult to maintain your calm, getting angry will not help the situation.

Given the importance of a dog's canine companions, it speaks volumes about the dog's adaptability as a species that we can

Ailments, Conditions, and Other Issues

condition them to accept being left alone at all! We're lucky we don't have far more problems than we do, especially in today's world, where few households have someone at home regularly during the day to keep the dog company.

Some behavior scientists theorize that experiencing a fear-causing event when a young dog is already mildly stressed about being alone can trigger more intense "home alone" anxiety behaviors. In addition, many of our pets are rescued from a neglected or negative environment, and these pets may have suffered tragic circumstances and, therefore, lack a sense of security and confidence.

Consult your veterinarian to make sure there is no underlying health issue that may be contributing to your dog's behavior. Ask your veterinarian or animal community for a recommendation for a credentialed animal behaviorist. In extreme cases, your veterinarian may recommend medication.

Here are some steps you can take to decrease your dog's anxious behavior. Walk your dog for 20–30 minutes prior to leaving your home. Make your departures and arrivals uneventful. Since your pet will miss you, it is best to limit the amount of petting, kisses and conversation prior to saying goodbye and when you return. This may be unnatural to you and even cold, but it is best to be a little neutral to minimize your pet's fear of your absence. Provide your pet with treats, chews and toys to keep their mouth and mind busy. Physical exercise and mental stimulation will calm your dog and make them more content. If you will be gone for several hours, consider hiring a dog walker or a dog sitter to keep your dog company during your absence.

Calm and soothe your pet with essential oils. Applying or diffusing lavender has been shown to inexpensively, safely and effectively reduce pet anxiety. Lavender combined with other essential oils offers pets greater support. For optimum impact diffuse Lavender with one of the following: Restful Blend, Comforting Blend,

Grounding Blend, Reassuring Blend and/or Frankincense in the home for 30–60 minutes prior to departure. An additional option is a pet collar diffuser. Depending on the length of time you will be gone and the degree of anxiety, some pets may need reapplication of essential oil(s) periodically. In this case, you could as your dog sitter to reapply the oils as needed.

Does your pet have a favorite blanket, bed or toy? Place a few drops of Restful Blend, Comforting blend, Reassuring Blend, Grounding Blend and/or Lavender on the object to comfort your pet. Apply on yourself the same essential oil you are using to calm your pet and act as a human diffuser. The pet will associate the aroma with you and will feel calmer and more secure.

An oral supplement of Copaiba offers powerful antioxidants, neurological support and helps to relieve anxiety. Continue to support overall health by feeding a high quality diet and supplementing with omega-3 and probiotics. The use of probiotics have been found to reduce anxiety in dogs, particularly by reducing the stress hormone cortisol (See Anxiety).

> *"After years of having a dog, you know him. You know the meaning of his snuffs and grunts and barks. Every twitch of the ears is a question or statement, every wag of the tail is an exclamation."*
>
> — Robert McCammon

Ailments, Conditions, and Other Issues

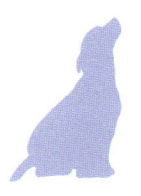

FOR DOGS

Apply 1 drop Lavender with 1 drop of either Restful Blend, Comforting Blend, Grounding Blend, Reassuring Blend and/or Frankincense diluted in 1 tsp. carrier oil for dogs.

Diffuse Lavender with either Restful Blend, Comforting Blend, Grounding Blend, Reassuring Blend or Frankincense prior to a leaving.

Apply 1-2 drops Lavender, Frankincense, Restful Blend, Comforting Blend, Grounding Blend, or Reassuring Blend on your pet's blanket, bed or toy.

Administer 1 Copaiba Softgel (for dogs over 30 lbs) 1-2 times daily. For smaller dogs, insert a toothpick in the regulator cap of Copaiba and add this amount of oil to the food 1-2 times daily. Administer 1 Restful Blend Softgel (for dogs over 15 lbs) 1-2 times daily (Restful Blend oil should not be given orally).

Feed a high quality diet supplemented with omega-3 and probiotics.

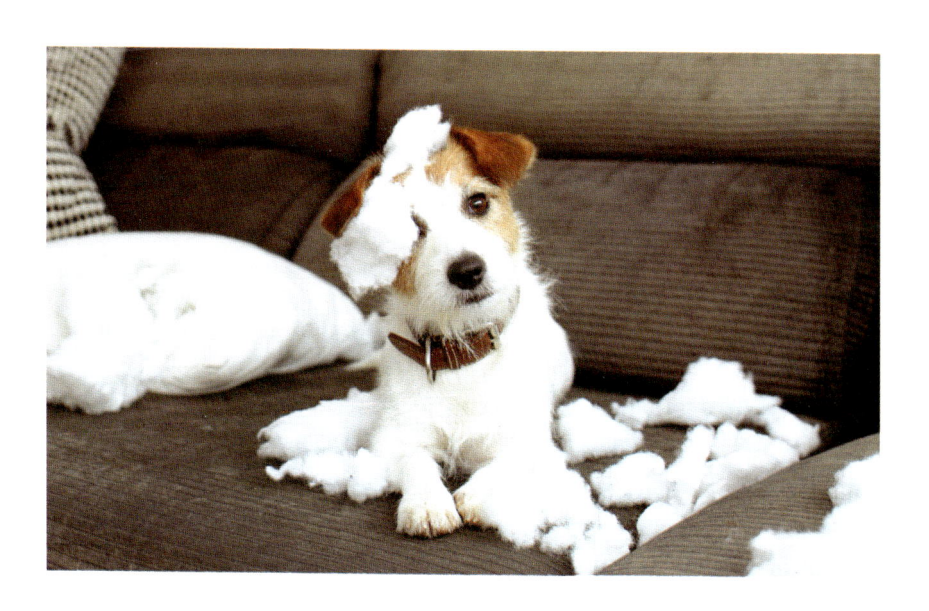

SNAKE BITES

Most snakes are not poisonous, but there are a few that cause concern. Snake bites are much more common in dogs than cats. In North America, there are about 25 species of venomous snakes. Some common venomous snakes are the Rattlesnake, Copperhead, Water Moccasin and Coral Snake. If bitten by any snake, take your pet to the veterinarian immediately. Even a non-poisonous snake bite can cause infection and an allergic reaction (See Cuts and Scrapes, Trauma, and Allergies).

A snake bite is an emergency. Antivenin needs to be administered as soon as possible to minimize the extent of the injury and help the dog recover. Your veterinarian can also care for your dog to prevent infection and complications.

Signs of a snake bite include redness, pain and inflammation at the site of the bite, lethargy, weakness, difficulty breathing, salivation, nausea and bruising of the skin and gums. If you suspect a snake bite, seek medical attention immediately.

Steps for Snakebite:
1. Take your pet to the veterinarian immediately. It is best to carry your dog rather than allow him or her to walk.
2. Stop any bleeding and immobilize the limb if possible. Keep the area bitten at or below the level of the heart.
3. Do not apply ice on the bite.
4. Clean the area carefully and cover if time permits.
5. Take a photo, if possible, and note the time of the bite.
6. Keep yourself and your pet calm.

Immediately apply Basil and one or more of the following: Myrrh, Lavender or Thyme. If you live in an area where poisonous snakes are common, add the above oils to your pet First Aid kit (See First Aid). After your pet has seen the veterinarian and received anti-venom treatment, apply Frankincense, Turmeric and Helichrysum (not recommended in deep puncture wounds) to speed healing. Administer an oral preparation of Copaiba to support the immune system and reduce inflammation. Diffuse and/or apply one of the following: Grounding Blend, Restful Blend, Reassuring Blend, Comforting Blend or Lavender to help keep you and your pet calm. Diffuse Protective Blend to support the immune system.

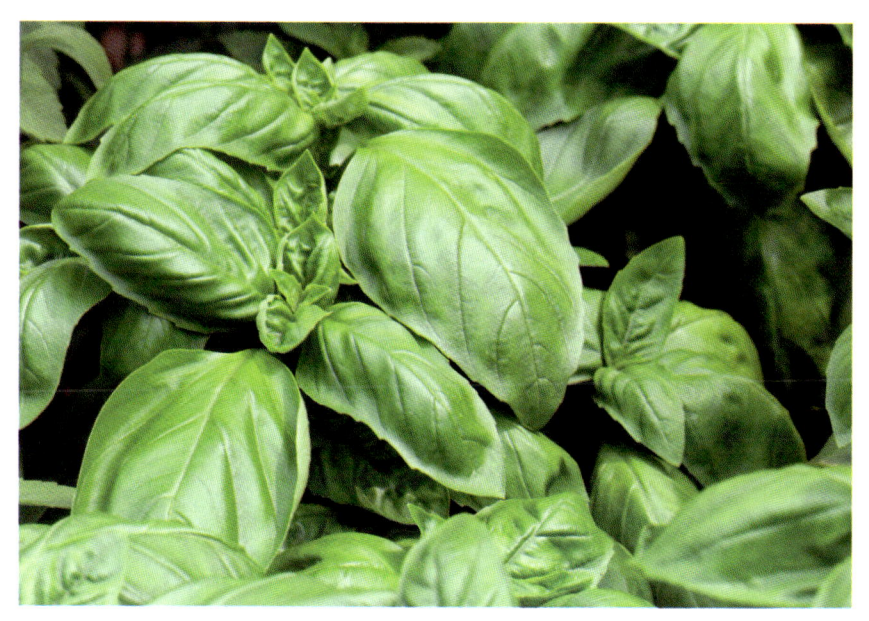

Basil

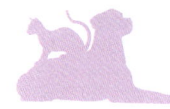

FOR DOGS & CATS

🛍️ Seek veterinary care immediately.

Apply 1 drop each Basil and one or more of the following: Myrrh, Lavender or Thyme diluted in 1 tsp. carrier oil (as soon as possible after the snake bite). Repeat every 2 hours until your pet has received medical attention.

After your pet has seen the veterinarian, apply 1 drop each Frankincense, Turmeric and Helichrysum diluted in 1 tsp. carrier oil 2–3 times daily or more if needed.

Apply 1 drop of Restful Blend, Comforting Blend or Lavender diluted in 1 tsp. carrier oil 2–3 times daily or more if needed.

Administer 1 Copaiba Softgel (for dogs over 30 lbs.) 1–2 times daily. For smaller dogs, insert a toothpick in the regulator cap of Copaiba and add this amount of oil to the food 1–2 times daily.

Diffuse Protective Blend for at least 20–30 minutes 2–3 times daily.

Diffuse Grounding Blend, Reassuring Blend or Lavender for at least 20–30 minutes 2–3 times daily.

SOUND SENSITIVITY

Loud sounds can be distressing to our pets. Stormy weather such as thunderstorms, heavy rain and high winds, and noises coming from fireworks and construction equipment can be upsetting to our pets. During certain times of the year, such as the summer, severe weather, thunderstorms and fireworks can be a common occurrence. For July 4th, what used to be a single celebration has evolved into a week long display of parades and fireworks in various surrounding towns. While families and children may enjoy the festivities, our pets often do not.

Many dogs and cats are quite fearful of these loud noises. Some dogs are so nervous that they hide, shake, soil in the home and become destructive to themselves or their homes. Cats tend to hide and isolate themselves in fear. It is saddening to see our pets suffer this way (See Anxiety and Stress).

Our pets sense our energy and emotions, our calm demeanor projects comfort to our pets. Reassure your pet, but not to the extent of coddling so as not to encourage fearful behavior. Be confident, relaxed and minimize the disturbances outside. Walking dogs for exercise is, of course, always beneficial but letting them be still and sniff to their heart's content is very calming and joyous for them. This can help to relax your dog.

Take the time before a holiday or event to let your dog sniff and smell the outdoors.

A busy pet will help him or her to be less sensitive to loud noises. Engage your cat in play time. Cats love to fetch, play with cat toys, chase a flashlight, and play find the treat. Chewing can help your dog to expend energy, so offering them hard rubber toys or bones could serve as a good distraction. Some of these can be stuffed with peanut butter, cream cheese, yogurt, or raw-food and frozen. Give them to your dog during the fireworks to keep them occupied.

Music is soothing to the savage beast. Canine music therapy can help provide balance. Classical music has been proven to calm dogs. We recommend using music which is created in a passive hearing mode rather than active listening. Passive hearing techniques facilitate relaxation. Soft music is not only calming for the dogs and cats, but equally relaxing and enjoyable for people. Sound is a potent energy that is not to be taken for granted – it has profound effects on all species.

Essential oils can be soothing to both your pets and you. We suggest applying and diffusing essential oils hours prior to the onset of a storm or a few days prior to fireworks. For mildly anxious dogs and cats, apply and diffuse Restful Blend or Lavender and Grounding blend. Moderately nervous pets may benefit from the addition of Frankincense and Copaiba or Vetiver. Some other suggestions include Reassuring Blend and Comforting Blend. For cats, add Lavender, Copaiba and Frankincense to the litter box (See Recipes: Litter Box Power). Those dogs who are severely afflicted may benefit from oral preparations of Copaiba and Restful blend. An oral supplement of Copaiba offers powerful antioxidants, neurological support and helps to relieve anxiety. Continue to support overall health by feeding a high quality diet and supplementing with omega-3 and probiotics. The use of probiotics have been found to reduce anxiety in pets, particularly by reducing the stress hormone cortisol. In the most extreme cases, a prescription medication may be needed as well.

"Everything I know I learned from dogs."
- Nora Roberts

Ailments, Conditions, and Other Issues

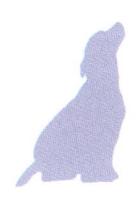

FOR DOGS

Apply 1 drop each Restful Blend and Grounding Blend in 1 tsp. carrier oil twice daily or more, if needed.

Diffuse Restful Blend and Grounding Blend for 20–30 minutes prior to and during a storm or stressful event.

Play soft music or a television program during an event.

For moderately nervous dogs, apply 1 drop each Restful Blend, Grounding Blend, Frankincense and Copaiba in 2 tsp. carrier oil twice daily or more if needed. For dogs with severe distress, add 1 drop Vetiver to this combination.

Administer 1 Copaiba Softgel (for dogs over 30 lbs.) 1–2 times daily. For smaller dogs, insert a toothpick in the regulator cap of Copaiba and add this amount of oil to the food 1–2 times daily. Administer 1 Restful Blend Softgel (for dogs over 15 lbs.) 1–2 times daily (Restful Blend oil should not be given orally).

Feed a high quality diet supplemented with omega-3 and probiotics.

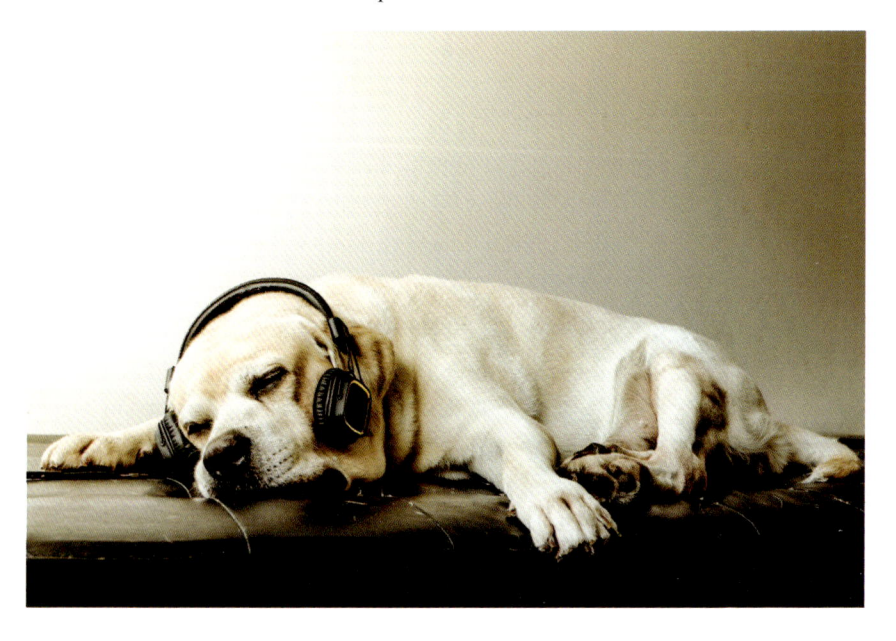

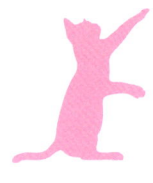

FOR CATS

Apply 1 drop each Restful Blend and Grounding Blend in 2 tsp. carrier oil twice daily or more, if needed.

Diffuse Restful Blend and Grounding Blend for 20–30 minutes prior to and during a storm or stressful event.

Play soft music or a television program during an event.

For moderately nervous cats, apply 1 drop each Restful Blend, Grounding Blend, Frankincense and Copaiba in 4 tsp. carrier oil twice daily or more if needed. For cats with severe distress, add 1 drop Vetiver to this combination.

Add 1 drop each Lavender, Copaiba and Frankincense to the litter box (See Recipes: Litter Box Power).

Feed a high quality diet supplemented with omega-3 and probiotics.

SPIDER BITES

Spiders have their place in the world, and we can certainly appreciate them for keeping away pests such as flies and mosquitos, but that doesn't mean you want them setting up camp in your bedroom or hiding out in your closet. There's no need to turn to insecticides or pesticides. Plenty of natural deterrents are available to keep spiders away from your home and your pets.

Spider bites can result in painful, red, swollen lesions or sores which may lead to infection. Avoid spiders by using Outdoor Blend (see Fleas, Ticks, and Mosquitoes) on your pet daily or as needed. In the event of a spider bite, directly apply Lavender and Basil which have anti-histaminic properties. Additionally, Lavender is very soothing, and Basil is a powerful pain reliever and helps to reduce swelling. Massage blend contains both Lavender and Basil and offers relief from itchy and painful bites.

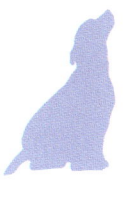

FOR DOGS

Apply 1 drop each Lavender and Basil or 1 drop Massage Blend in 1 tsp. carrier oil 2–3 times daily or more if needed.

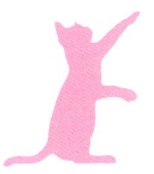

FOR CATS

Apply 1 drop each Lavender and Basil or 1 drop Massage Blend in 2 tsp. carrier oil 2–3 times daily or more if needed.

Spider Control

Diffuse Outdoor Blend, Cleansing Blend, Peppermint or Lavender in areas of the home likely to attract spiders such as enclosed porches, basements and attics.

Spray areas in your home with Spider-Stay-Away-Spray. Before using the spray, vacuum any egg sacs or old spider webs using the hose attachment and dispose of the contents properly.

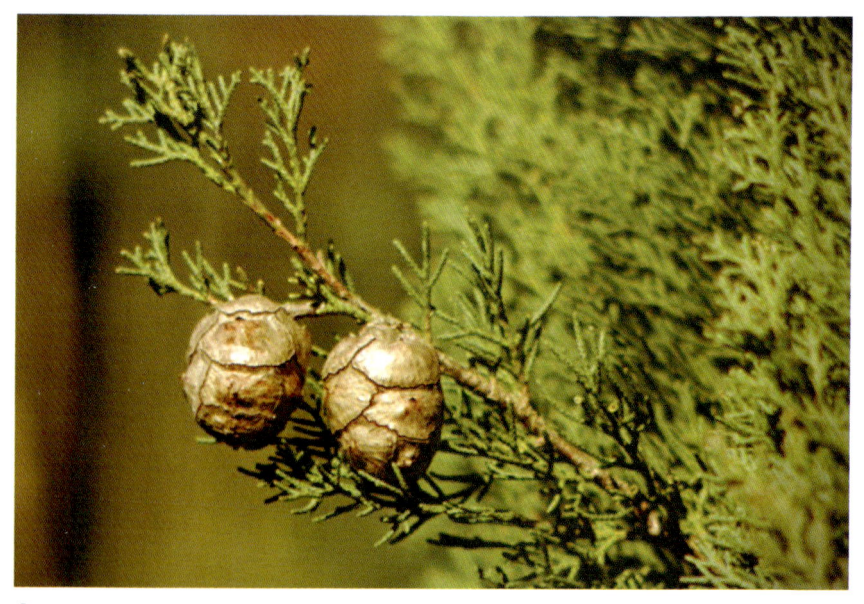

Cypress

Natural Spider-Stay-Away-Spray

Ingredients

16 oz. warm water
1 Tbsp. liquid dish soap
1 Tbsp. white vinegar (optional)
5–7 drops Peppermint Essential Oil
5–7 drops Melaleuca Essential Oil
5–7 drops Lavender Essential Oil
Glass or Plastic Spray Bottle*

Instructions

Put 5–7 drops of each essential oil in an empty glass or plastic spray bottle and fill mostly to the top with warm water. Add 1 tablespoon of natural dish soap, replace the top. Shake the bottle well before use. Spray the corners of window frames, along door cracks, or in dark, dingy places spiders may be hiding out. You may also add a teaspoon of white vinegar to the mixture, but keep in mind that vinegar may affect some fabrics and surfaces.

TICK-BORNE DISEASES

Ticks are present throughout the United States and may be infected with bacteria, viruses and parasites. Ticks tend to bite dogs more commonly than cats. Some of the diseases that Ticks may carry are Lyme, Ehrlichiosis, Rocky Mountain Spotted Fever, Anaplasmosis, Tick Paralysis and Cytauxzoonosis. This is just a small representation of the more than dozen illnesses that are carried by ticks. Most of these diseases may also be transferred to people via a tick bite. Lyme disease is the most commonly reported tick-borne disease in the United States. The reported cases of Lyme disease has doubled in the United States over the last 10 years. The reason for the increase in tick-borne illnesses is unclear, as a number of factors can affect tick numbers each year, including temperature, rainfall, humidity and host populations such as mice, deer and other animals. Pets may be inflicted with more than one disease at the same time and may get a tick borne illness multiple times throughout their life. For these reasons, good tick control is crucial in protecting your pet from the possible acquisition of these dangerous diseases.

Keeping your pet healthy, with a strong immune system, will help reduce the severity of illness and decrease the possibility of long term chronic symptoms and ailments. It has been found, that dogs infected with Lyme disease have an increased likelihood of developing kidney disease later in life (See Organ Support), joint pain (See Pain and Arthritis) and autoimmune disease (See Autoimmune Disease), even if they have successfully completed treatment.

If you find a tick on your pet, you (or your veterinarian) may remove it by tweezing around it, as close to the skin as possible. Do not squeeze the tick's body. In removing the entire tick, you may take away some of your dog's skin, since the tick is firmly attached. The skin will heal, and removing a small amount of skin will ensure

Ailments, Conditions, and Other Issues

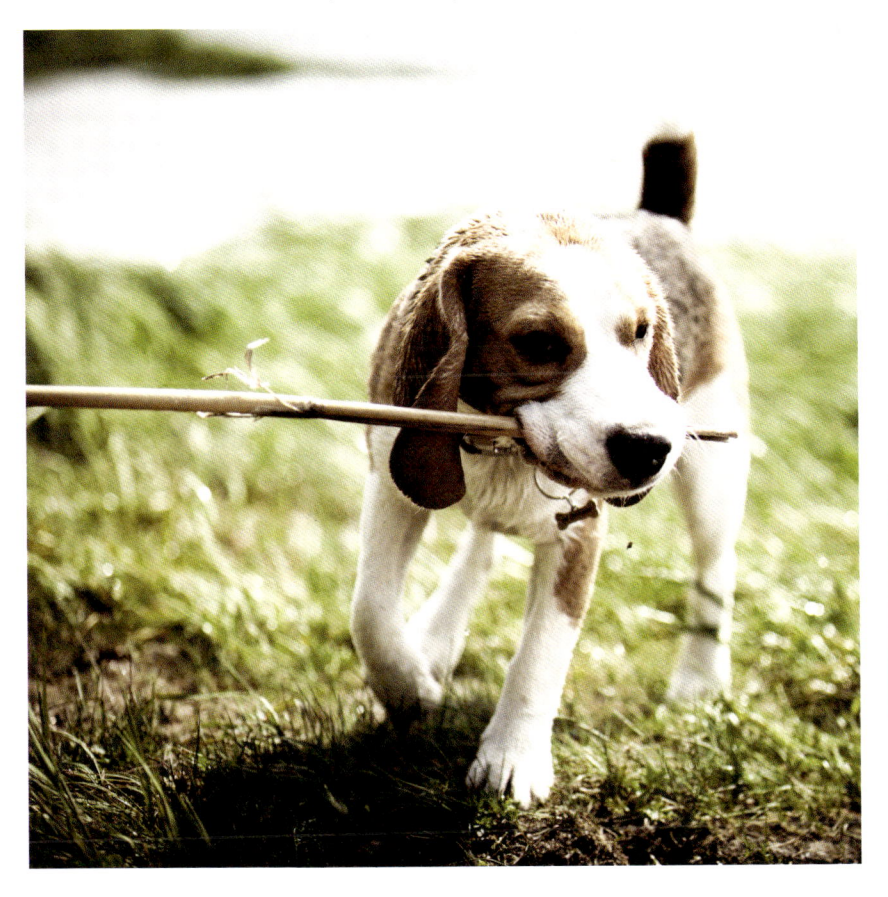

that the entire tick has been extracted. In either case, whether you remove the tick or not, call your veterinarian.

If your dog has contracted a disease from the tick, signs may not be noticed for several days to weeks. Some common symptoms your pet may exhibit are lethargy, depression, joint pain, reduced activity, decreased appetite, fever, incoordination or pale gums. Monitor your pet closely for any of these symptoms, which may not be noticed for several days to weeks. At any sign of illness, call your veterinarian for a physical exam and appropriate diagnostic testing.

Tick-borne diseases are generally treated with antibiotics. Use essential oils to complement traditional therapy. We suggest two combinations of essential oils: one to eradicate infection and the other to support the immune system. Apply directly to the site of the tick bite a combination of Thyme, Geranium and Arborvitae daily. To support the immune system, apply a combination of Lavender, Myrrh and Helichrysum daily. After treatment is completed and to prevent possible long term consequences, apply Frankincense and Juniper Berry daily (See Longevity: A Long and Healthy Life).

To support the immune, system administer 1 Copaiba Softgel (for dogs over 30 lbs.) 1–2 times daily. For smaller dogs, insert a toothpick in the regulator cap of Copaiba and add this amount of oil to the food 1–2 times daily.

Feed your pet a high quality diet and supplement with Omega-3 and probiotics.

For ongoing protection, bathe your pet with natural Flea and Tick Shampoo, and apply natural Flea and Tick Repellant Spray (see Fleas, Ticks and Mosquitoes) daily or as needed.

> *"Dogs are our link to paradise. They don't know evil or jealousy or discontent."*
>
> — Milan Kundera

Ailments, Conditions, and Other Issues

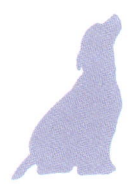

FOR DOGS

Seek veterinary care immediately.

Remove the tick with tweezers very close to the skin. Do not squeeze the tick's body.

Apply 1 drop each of Thyme, Geranium and Arborvitae in 1 tsp. carrier oil for dogs and 2 tsp. carrier oil for puppies (less than 4 months) to the area of the tick bite 2–3 times daily or more if needed.

Apply 1 drop each Lavender ,Myrrh and Helichrysum in 1 tsp. carrier oil for dogs and 2 tsp. carrier oil for puppies (less than 4 months) 2–3 times daily or more if needed.

Administer 1 Copaiba Softgel (for dogs over 30 lbs.) 1–2 times daily for dogs. For smaller dogs, insert a toothpick in the regulator cap of Copaiba and add this amount of oil to the food 1–2 times daily.

Post treatment: Apply 1 drop each Frankincense and Juniper Berry in 1 tsp. carrier oil for dogs and 2 tsp. carrier oil for puppies (less than 4 months) daily for your dog's life.

Bathe your pet with natural Flea and Tick Shampoo, and apply natural Flea and Tick Repellant Spray (see Fleas, Ticks and Mosquitoes) daily or as needed.

Feed your pet a high quality diet and supplement with Omega-3 and probiotics.

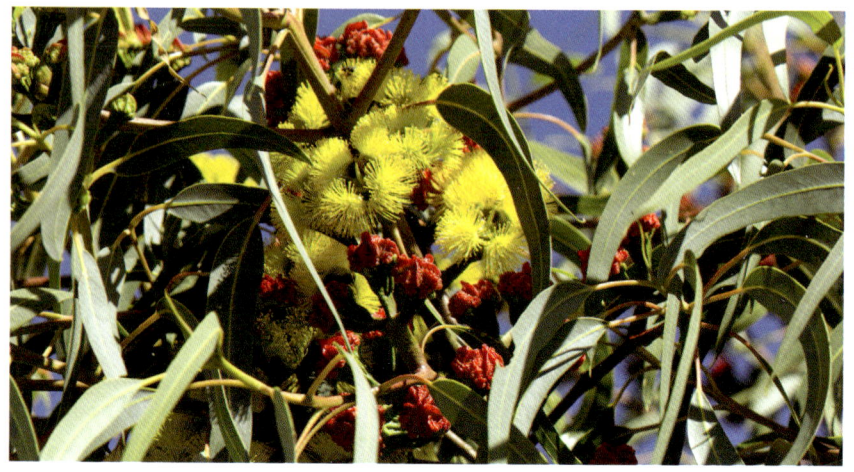

Eucalyptus

Homemade Flea and Tick Collar

Ingredients

5 drops Eucalyptus Essential Oil
5 drops Geranium Essential oil
5 drops Thyme Essential Oil
5 drops Lemongrass Essential Oil
5 drops Repellant Essential Oil Blend
4 oz. distilled water
Glass or Plastic Container*
For puppies younger than 4 months or for dogs weighing less than 15 pounds, use 2 drops of each recommended essential oil in 8 oz. of distilled water.
For cats, use 1 drop each Arborvitae, Geranium, Thyme, Lemongrass, and Repellant Blend in 8 oz. of distilled water.

Instructions

Mix distilled water with the essential oils in a glass or plastic container. Soak a nylon/cloth collar in the solution for 20 minutes.
Remove collar and allow it to dry thoroughly before placing it on your pet. Re-soak the collar every two weeks or more frequently as needed.

> *"Animals know that the ultimate point of life is to enjoy it."*
>
> — Samuel Butler

Flea & Tick Repellent Shampoo or Spray

Ingredients
8 oz. Natural Shampoo Base or Water
4 drops Clary Sage Essential Oil
2 drops Cleansing Essential Oil Blend
5 drops Repellant Essential Oil Blend
8 drops Peppermint Essential Oil
4 drops Lemon Essential Oil
2 drops Geranium Essential Oil
2 drops Eucalyptus Essential Oil
3 drops Lavender Essential Oil
2 drops Myrrh Essential Oil
2 drops Thyme Essential Oil
Glass or Plastic Bottle*

Instructions:
Add essential oils to an empty glass or plastic bottle. Top with water. Shake the bottle well before use. Spray your pet, bedding and yourself!

TRAUMA

In the event your pet suffers a severe injury, fall, bleeding, fire, a fight with another animal or is hit by a car, contact your veterinarian or an animal emergency facility immediately. If you have help, begin supporting your pet and yourself with essential oils. The following recommendations for injuries may be implemented immediately following the injury and continued after your pet has seen the veterinarian. In every traumatic situation, diffusing essential oils is beneficial.

If your pet has an open wound (See Cuts and Scrapes): Apply pressure to stop any bleeding and immobilize your pet. Apply Helichrysum (do not use if it is a puncture wound) and Cypress essential oils to help stop the bleeding (See Healing Salve, Healing Spray and Healing Oil Blend recipes below) and Lavender to reduce pain (See Pain). We suggest diffusing a combination of Helichrysum, Renewing Blend, Frankincense, Cedarwood and Lavender.

If your pet has suffered a fall or has been hit by a car: There is a possibility that your pet has suffered bruising, sprained a limb or broken a bone (See Broken Bones). Apply Frankincense, Grounding Blend, Massage Blend, Lavender and Copaiba to reduce pain, inflammation, bruising and swelling. We suggest diffusing a combination of Ginger, Renewing Blend, Frankincense, Cedarwood and Lavender.

If your pet gets into a fight with another animal: Take care when you are breaking up a fight not to get bitten. Apply pressure to stop any bleeding and immobilize the area. Use Cypress, Lavender, Copaiba and Frankincense to reduce swelling, bruising, possible infection and tissue damage. We suggest diffusing a combination of Copaiba, Renewing Blend, Frankincense, Cedarwood and Lavender.

Ailments, Conditions, and Other Issues

If your pet is exposed to a fire: Check your pet for burns (See Burns; and See Healing Salve, Healing Spray and Healing Oil Blend recipes below) and help support your pet's respiratory and cardiovascular systems (See Respiratory Conditions, Organ Support). Apply Lavender and Helichrysum to soothe the burn. Apply Respiratory Blend alternating with Renewing Blend and Frankincense to support and strengthen the lungs and promote easeful breathing. Diffuse Respiratory Blend or Renewing Blend and add Protective Blend and Frankincense to support the heart and lungs.

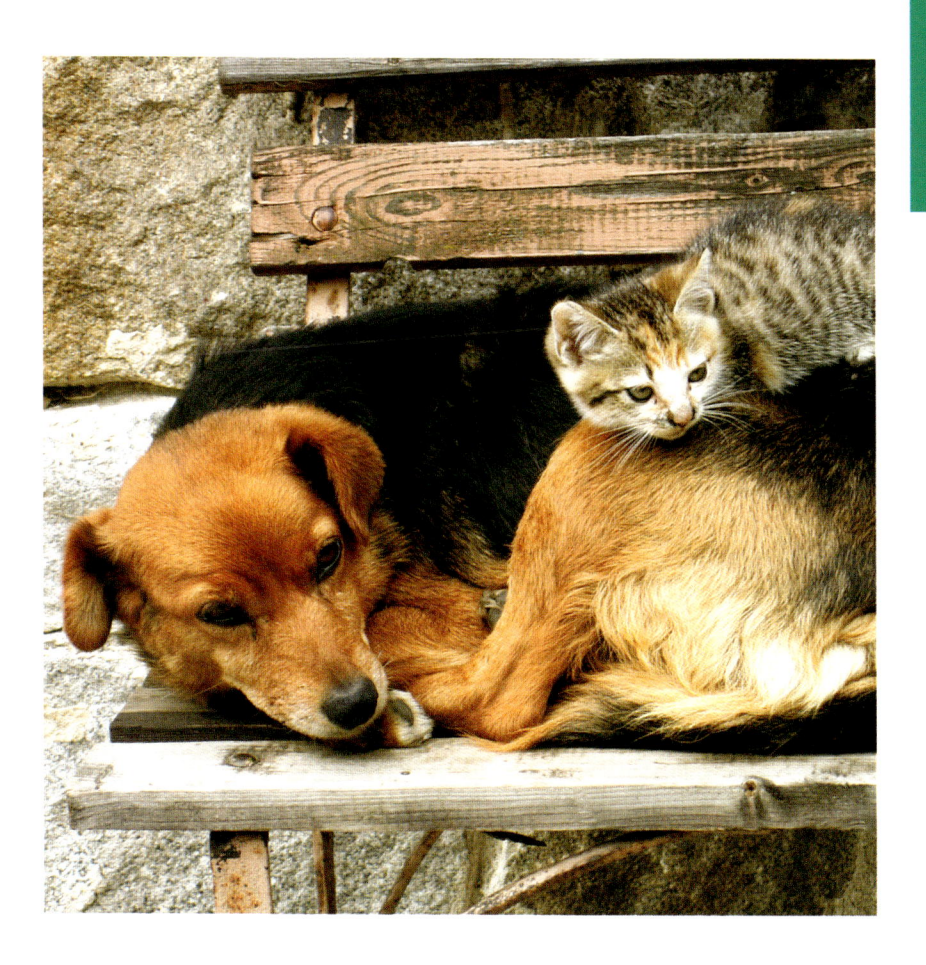

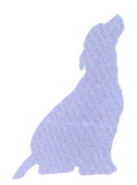

FOR DOGS

Seek veterinary care immediately.

Wounds: Soak a gauze pad or soft cloth in 1 cup of warm water containing 1 drop each Helichrysum, Lavender and Cypress and apply to the wound.

Apply 1 drop each Lavender, Helichrysum and Cypress in 1 tsp. carrier oil 2–3 times daily or more if needed.

Diffuse two of the following essential oils: Helichrysum, Renewing Blend, Frankincense, Cedarwood or Lavender for 20–30 minutes 2–3 times daily.

Fall or Car Accident: Apply 1 drop each Frankincense, Grounding Blend, Massage Blend, Lavender and Copaiba in 2 tsp. carrier oil 2–3 times daily or more if needed.

Diffuse Ginger and Frankincense for 20–30 minutes 2–3 times daily. One of the following oils, Renewing Blend, Cedarwood and Lavender, may be added to the above combination.

Animal Fight: Apply pressure to stop any bleeding and immobilize the area.

Apply 1 drop each Cypress, Lavender, Copaiba and Frankincense in 1 tsp. carrier oil 2–3 times daily or more if needed.

Diffuse two or three of the following essential oils: Copaiba, Renewing Blend, Frankincense, Cedarwood or Lavender for 20–30 minutes 2–3 times daily.

Fire: To the burn, apply 1 drop each Lavender and Helichrysum in 1 tsp. Aloe Vera Gel 3–4 times daily.

For smoke inhalation, apply 1 drop each Respiratory Blend and Frankincense alternating daily with 1 drop each Renewing Blend and Frankincense in 2 tsp. carrier oil 3–4 times daily.

Ailments, Conditions, and Other Issues

Diffuse Respiratory Blend alternating with Renewing Blend. Combine one of the two previous oils with Protective Blend and Frankincense for 30–60 minutes 2–3 times daily or more if needed. If your pet has suffered lung trauma, you may choose to use a tent or confine your pet to one room while diffusing. If you confine your pet to one room, we recommend monitoring your pet for safety.

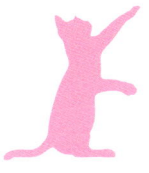

FOR CATS

Seek veterinary care immediately.

Wounds: Soak a gauze pad or soft cloth in 1 cup of warm water containing 1 drop each Helichrysum, Lavender and Cypress and apply to the wound.

Apply 1 drop each Lavender, Helichrysum and Cypress in 2 tsp. carrier oil 2–3 times daily or more if needed.

Diffuse two of the following essential oils: Helichrysum, Renewing Blend, Frankincense, Cedarwood or Lavender for 20–30 minutes 2–3 times daily.

Fall or Car Accident: Apply 1 drop each Frankincense, Grounding Blend, Massage Blend, Lavender and Copaiba in 4 tsp. carrier oil 2–3 times daily or more if needed.

Diffuse Ginger and Frankincense for 20–30 minutes 2–3 times daily. One of the following oils, Renewing Blend, Cedarwood and Lavender, may be added to the above combination.

Animal Fight: Apply pressure to stop any bleeding and immobilize the area.

Apply 1 drop each Cypress, Lavender, Copaiba and Frankincense in 2 tsp. carrier oil 2–3 times daily or more if needed.

Diffuse two or three of the following essential oils: Copaiba, Renewing Blend, Frankincense, Cedarwood or Lavender for 20–30 minutes 2–3 times daily.

Fire: To the burn, apply 1 drop each Lavender and Helichrysum in 1 tsp. Aloe Vera Gel 3-4 times daily.

For smoke inhalation, apply 1 drop each Respiratory Blend and Frankincense alternating daily with 1 drop each Renewing Blend and Frankincense in 4 tsp. carrier oil 3-4 times daily.

Diffuse Respiratory Blend alternating with Renewing Blend. Combine one of the two previous oils with Protective Blend and Frankincense for 30-60 minutes 2-3 times daily or more if needed. If your pet has suffered lung trauma, you may choose to use a tent or confine your pet to one room while diffusing. If you confine your pet to one room, we recommend monitoring your pet for safety.

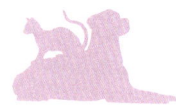

FOR DOGS & CATS

If your pet has suffered lung trauma, you may choose to use a tent or confine your pet to one room while diffusing. If you confine your pet to one room, we recommend monitoring your pet for safety (See How to Use Essential Oils).

The result of trauma can be varied and can result in skin irritations and abrasions may occur. Follow the specific directions below and use Healing Salve, Healing Spray and Healing Oil Blend as needed.

Diffuse Respiratory Blend alternating with Renewing Blend. Combine one of the two previous oils with Protective Blend and Frankincense for 30-60 minutes 2-3 times daily or more if needed.

"When I am feeling low all I have to do is watch my cats and my courage returns."
- Charles Bukowski

Healing Spray/Healing Oil Blend

Ingredients
5 drops Frankincense Essential Oil
5 drops Geranium Essential Oil
5 drops Lavender Essential Oil
5 drops Helichrysum Essential Oil
5 drops Myrrh Essential Oil
4 oz. water or Aloe Vera Juice for the spray
    OR
3–4 tsp. carrier oil such as Fractionated Coconut Oil
For dogs only: *If no relief is noted in 24 hours, add 5 drops of Arborvitae to the Healing Spray and Healing Oil Blend.*
4 oz. Glass or Plastic Spray Bottle*

Instructions
Add essential oils to glass or plastic spray bottle. Top with water, Aloe Vera Juice or Carrier Oil. Shake the bottle well before use.

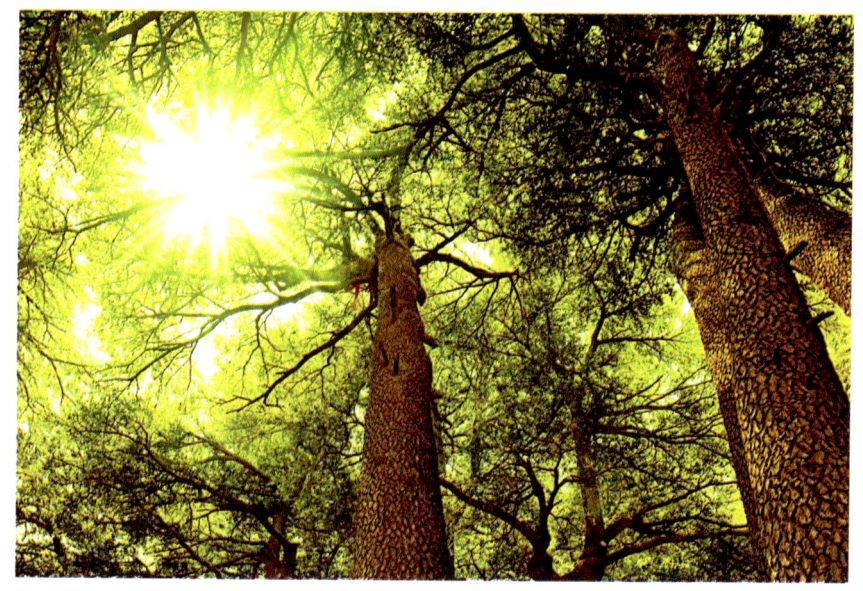

Cedarwood

Ailments, Conditions, and Other Issues

Healing Salve

Ingredients
8 ounces Cold-Pressed Organic Coconut Oil
1 ounce Beeswax
2 drops Vitamin E (optional)
10 drops Lavender Essential Oil
5 drops Myrrh Essential Oil
3 drops Helichrysum Essential Oil
Glass Jars or Tin Containers

Place the coconut oil and beeswax over a double –boiler, and gently warm over low heat until the beeswax melts. Remove from heat and add the essential oils and Vitamin E oil, (if using). Quickly pour the mixture into glass jars or tins, and allow to cool completely. Store salve in a cool location where they will not re-melt and re-solidify. When stored correctly, salve will last for 1–3 years. Yields 8 ounces.

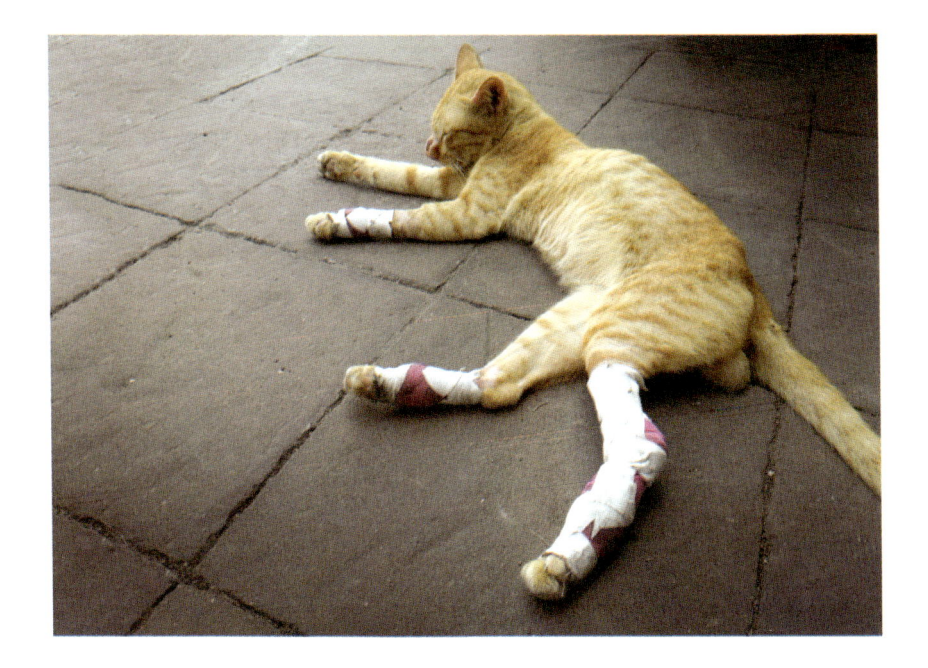

URINARY BLOCKAGE (PRIMARILY MALE CATS)

A urinary blockage or the inability to urinate is an emergency. If your cat has not urinated in 12–24 hours, contact your veterinarian.

Male cats are more prone to urinary blockage due to the small size (diameter) of the urethra. The blockage is due to crystals, sand or minerals that form as a result of your cat's diet and accumulate in the narrow urethra. Some signs of urinary blockage might be frequent visits to the litter box, straining to urinate, and vocalizing in the litter box, which is an indication of pain or discomfort. Even though your cat may visit the litter box, the litter box may be dry or have only small drips of urine. The inability to urinate leads to an accumulation of toxins in the body. This condition is serious and can have detrimental effects on your cat's kidneys and may even result in death (See Urinary Conditions and Organ Support).

Treatment usually involves hospitalization to relieve the blockage, address inflammation and potential infection. Some cats suffer repeated urinary blockages and may require surgery to eliminate the possibility of a recurrence. Poor quality pet food is a primary cause of this condition. We suggest speaking to your veterinarian or nutritionist about possible diet changes.

To complement veterinary care, apply diluted Juniper Berry, Lemongrass, Copaiba, Cypress and Geranium. These oils help to reduce inflammation, act as a diuretic, and have cleansing and purifying qualities. For pain, apply Massage Blend and Lavender. Add Juniper Berry, Ylang Ylang, and Lavender to the litter box as described in Litter Box Power (See Recipes: Litter Box Power). Diffuse Protective Blend or Juniper Berry to help decrease toxins and support the immune system. Feed an appropriate diet guided by you veterinarian and supplement with Omega-3 and probiotics.

Ailments, Conditions, and Other Issues

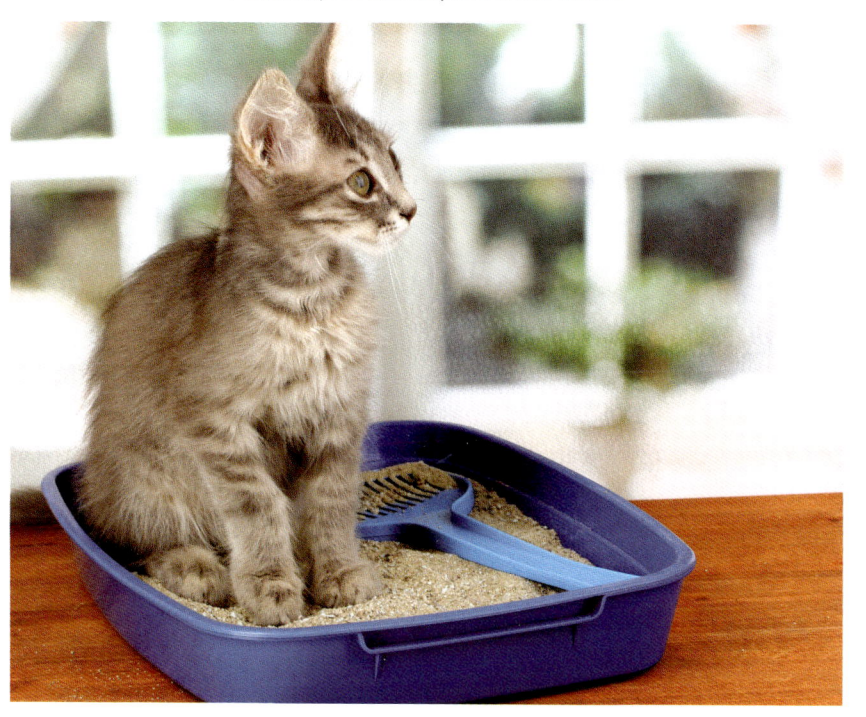

"Cats are furry waterfalls of grace"
— Layla Morgan Wilde

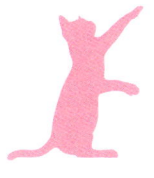

FOR CATS

Seek veterinary care immediately.

Apply 1 drop each Juniper Berry, Lemongrass, Copaiba, Cypress, and Geranium diluted in 4 tsp. carrier oil twice daily.

Apply 1 drop each Massage Blend and Lavender in 2 tsp. carrier oil twice daily as needed for discomfort.

Add Juniper Berry, Ylang Ylang, and Lavender to the litter box as described in Litter Box Power (See Recipes: Litter Box Power).

URINARY CONDITIONS

Both dogs and cats may develop changes in urinary habits and any change may indicate an underlying problem. Some signs include increased frequency of urination, straining to urinate, squatting frequently, scooting, licking the genitalia, urinary accidents in the home or, for cats, urinating outside the litter box. Sometimes, the urine is visibly discolored or bloody. Older pets often develop incontinence, loss of urine or loss of control of their bladder in which they may be unaware that they are urinating. Owners often discover puddles or wet areas where the pet has been sleeping or resting (See Canine Cognitive Disorder).

Similar symptoms may be present for a number of urinary conditions including bladder infections, urinary tract infections (UTI), bladder stones or crystals, kidney disease and cancer (See Organ Support, Urinary Blockage, Diabetes and Cancer). It is best to see your veterinarian for an examination and appropriate diagnostic testing and treatment. Often, infections of the urinary system require medication. Bladder stones generally require surgical removal. Both conditions benefit from changes in nutrition, supplements and probiotics. Proper hydration is very important in clearing infection and toxins from the body and in promoting a healthy urinary system.

Essential oils complement traditional therapy and support a strong immune system and nervous system. Assist your pet's urinary system with Juniper Berry, Lemongrass, Cypress and Geranium. These oils help to reduce inflammation, act as a diuretic, and have cleansing and purifying qualities. For pain, apply Massage Blend and Lavender. Some pets suffer from chronic UTIs. Some common causes of recurring infections are drug resistant bacteria, underlying metabolic disease, stress, and anxiety. In these cases, we suggest alternating between the following two combinations: Juniper Berry,

Ailments, Conditions, and Other Issues

Lemongrass, Cypress and Geranium and Juniper Berry, Frankincense, Arborvitae, and Myrrh.

For dogs, administer an oral preparation of Copaiba for inflammation, pain relief and immune support. Diffuse Protective Blend or Juniper Berry to decrease toxins and support the immune system. Feed an appropriate diet guided by you veterinarian and supplement with Omega-3 and probiotics.

For cats, add Juniper Berry, Ylang Ylang, and Lavender to the litter box as described in Litter Box Power (See Recipes: Litter Box Power). Diffuse Protective Blend or Juniper Berry to decrease toxins and support the immune system. Feed an appropriate diet guided by your veterinarian and supplement with Omega-3 and probiotics.

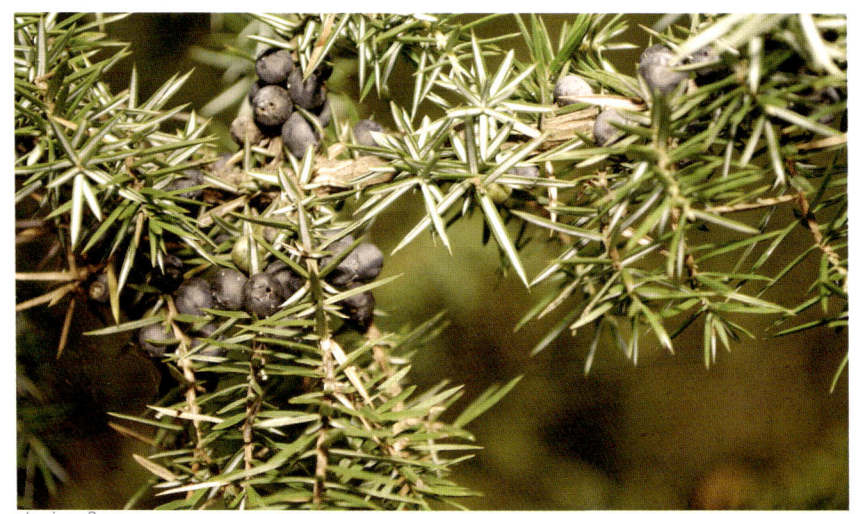

Juniper Berry

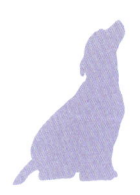

FOR DOGS

Apply 1 drop each Juniper Berry, Lemongrass, Cypress and Geranium diluted in 2 tsp. carrier oil twice daily.

Apply 1 drop each Massage Blend and Lavender in 1 tsp. carrier oil if indicated.

Administer 1 Copaiba Softgel (for dogs over 30 lbs.) 1–2 times daily. For smaller dogs, insert a toothpick in the regulator cap of Copaiba and add this amount of oil to the food 1–2 times daily. Diffuse Protective Blend or Juniper Berry for 20–30 minutes 2–3 times daily.

For Chronic UTIs: Follow the above directions. If your pet is diagnosed with a second infection, apply 1 drop each Juniper Berry, Frankincense, Arborvitae, and Myrrh diluted in 1 tsp. carrier oil twice daily.

Feed an appropriate diet guided by your veterinarian and supplement with Omega-3 and probiotics.

Ailments, Conditions, and Other Issues

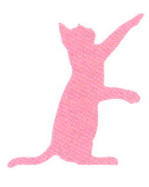

FOR CATS

Apply 1 drop each Juniper Berry, Lemongrass, Cypress and Geranium diluted in 4 tsp. carrier oil twice daily.

Apply 1 drop each Massage Blend and Lavender in 2 tsp. carrier oil if indicated.

Add Juniper Berry, Ylang Ylang, and Lavender to the litter box as described in Litter Box Power (See Recipes: Litter Box Power).

For Chronic UTIs: Follow the above directions. If your pet is diagnosed with a second infection, apply 1 drop each Juniper Berry, Frankincense, Arborvitae, and Myrrh diluted in 4 tsp. carrier oil twice daily.

Feed an appropriate diet guided by your veterinarian and supplement with Omega-3 and probiotics.

"There are few things in life more heartwarming than to be welcomed by a cat.

- Tay Hohoff

URINATING OUTSIDE OF THE LITTER BOX

Cats may refuse to use the litter box for a number of reasons. Some possible causes include painful urination such as a urinary tract infection (See Urinary Conditions). In other cases, your cat may be expressing his or her disapproval of the type of box, litter, location or cleanliness of the box. He or she may also be expressing feelings of stress, anger, grief or fear (See Anxiety and Stress, Grief). On some occasions, a cat may associate a negative event or noise with the litter box and, subsequently, avoid it. Another possibility is if your cat has urinated outside the box in a specific location in your home, it will return to that same location, often because of the lingering smell of urine. A rule of thumb is to provide one litter box per cat plus one extra. Scoop the boxes at least once daily. Fully clean the boxes and change the litter weekly. Clean any soiled areas in your home with vinegar and added essential oils (See Green Cleaning).

If your cat neglects to use the litter box for several days, visit your veterinarian for a thorough physical exam and appropriate diagnostic testing and medical treatment, if necessary.

Apply Lavender or Restful Blend to your cat daily for stress and anxiety. Diffuse Grounding Blend, Restful Blend, Reassuring Blend, or Comforting Blend for calming. For odor elimination, diffuse Rosemary, Lavender and Cedarwood or Cleansing Blend.

Add Grounding Blend, Restful Blend, Lavender or Cleansing Blend to the litter box as described in Litter Box Power. Clean your home with Protective Blend natural cleaner and clean any soiled areas with Hydrogen Peroxide, Vinegar, Baking Soda, and Wild Orange Oil.

Ailments, Conditions, and Other Issues

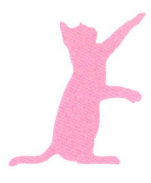

FOR CATS

Apply 1 drop Lavender or Restful Blend diluted in 2 tsp. carrier twice daily.

Diffuse Grounding Blend, Cleansing Blend, Restful Blend, Comforting Blend or Reassuring Blend for 20–30 minutes 2–3 times daily.

For Calming: Add 1 drop each Lavender, Copaiba and Roman Chamomile to the litter box (See Receipes: Litter Box Power).

For Kidney and Bladder Issues: Add 1 drop each Juniper Berry and Ylang Ylang or Lavender to the litter box.

For Odor Control: Add 2 drops Cleansing Blend or Rosemary to the litter box.

Clean with Protective Blend natural cleaner.

Spray soiled area with Hydrogen Peroxide, Vinegar, Baking Soda, and Wild Orange Oil.

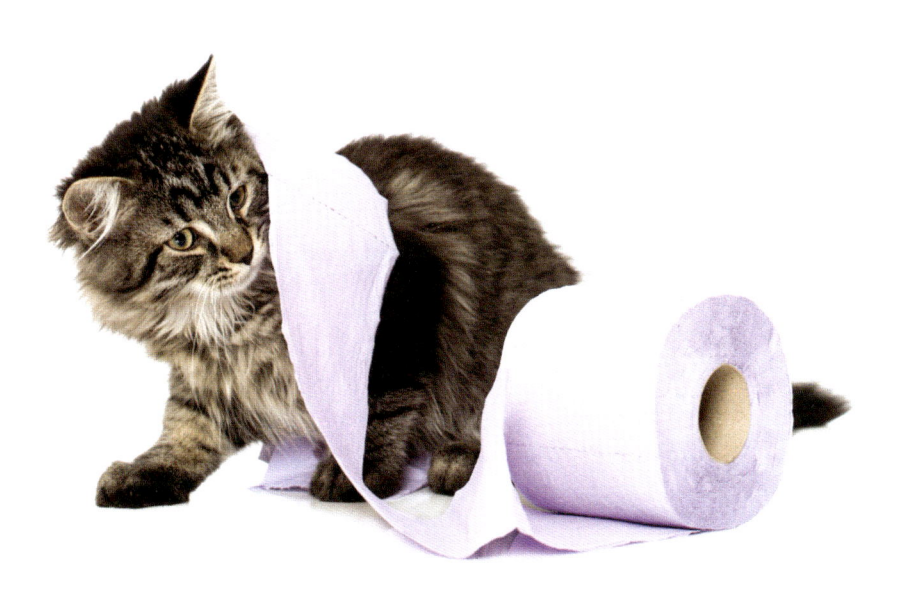

Urine Odor Eliminating Spray

Ingredients:
5 oz. Hydrogen Peroxide
1 tsp. Vinegar
1 tsp. Baking Soda
3 drops Wild Orange Essential Oil
Glass or Plastic Spray Bottle*

Instructions:
Add the essential oil to the empty bottle. Add the baking soda followed by the vinegar and hydrogen peroxide. Shake the bottle well before use. Now simply spray the affected area generously with the solution and allow to completely dry. It will become powder-like once the formula dries. Once it dries, vacuum up the powder.

If the smell remains, spray and vacuum again and follow with the powder described below.

VACCINE DETOXIFICATION

The purpose of a vaccination is to prepare the immune system to recognize a specific germ, so that your pet is protected if he or she is exposed to that bacteria or virus. The subject of vaccination is controversial, and much has been speculated about the dangers of vaccines on ourselves, our children and our pets. Vaccines contain numerous ingredients, some of which are preservatives, additives and heavy metals which may accumulate in the body. These metals may have deleterious effects on the body, and their full impact on overall health may not yet be known. We suggest you have a conversation with your veterinarian regarding vaccinating your pet. A vaccine protocol may be customized for your pet depending upon his or her individual lifestyle, where you live and the risk of exposure.

After your pet has been vaccinated, there are a number of options to help reduce the unnecessary components and contaminants of the vaccine. A probiotic supplement contains healthy bacteria that have been shown to help maintain an optimal digestive system and to remove toxins and other heavy metals from the body. The lymphatic system is the body's primary waste removal system, and Omega-3 fatty acids have been found to improve lymphatic flow, helping to eliminate toxins from the body and support the immune system. Omega-3 essential fatty acids are required for all functions of the liver including detoxification. For these reasons, we suggest feeding your pet a high quality diet supplemented with Omega-3 and probiotics.

Essential oils will help to prepare your pet's immune system and liver to receive and process a vaccination. Prior to vaccination, apply

SpOil Your Pet

Geranium, Helichrysum and Juniper Berry or Detoxification Blend. Apply Roman Chamomile around the injection site to decrease any localized skin irritation. Post vaccination, apply Helichrysum, Geranium, Roman Chamomile, Copaiba and Juniper Berry to help support the liver and immune system and aid in the elimination of any toxic ingredients. If your pet is experiencing discomfort and swelling after he or she is given a vaccine, add Frankincense or Massage Blend to the post vaccination oils listed above.

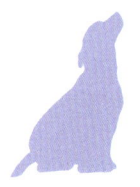

FOR DOGS

3–5 days prior to vaccination:
Apply 1 drop each Geranium, Helichrysum and Juniper Berry or Detoxification Blend in 2 tsp. carrier oil twice daily.

3–5 days post vaccination:
Apply 1 drop Roman Chamomile diluted in 1 tsp. carrier oil around the injection site twice daily or as needed.

Combine 1 drop each Helichrysum, Geranium and Juniper Berry or Detoxification Blend with 1 drop each Roman Chamomile and Copaiba in 2 tsp. carrier oil and apply twice daily.

For discomfort: Apply 1 drop Frankincense or Massage Blend in 1 tsp. carrier oil twice daily or as needed.

Feed your pet a high quality diet supplemented with Omega-3 and probiotics.

Ailments, Conditions, and Other Issues

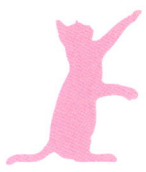

FOR CATS

3–5 days prior to vaccination:
Apply 1 drop each Geranium, Helichrysum and Juniper Berry or Detoxification Blend in 4 tsp. carrier oil twice daily.

3–5 days post vaccination:
Apply 1 drop Roman Chamomile diluted in 2 tsp. carrier oil around the injection site twice daily or as needed.

Combine 1 drop each Helichrysum, Geranium and Juniper Berry or Detoxification Blend with 1 drop each Roman Chamomile and Copaiba in 4 tsp. carrier oil and apply twice daily.

For discomfort: Apply 1 drop Frankincense or Massage Blend in 2 tsp. carrier oil twice daily or as needed.

Feed your pet a high quality diet supplemented with Omega-3 and probiotics.

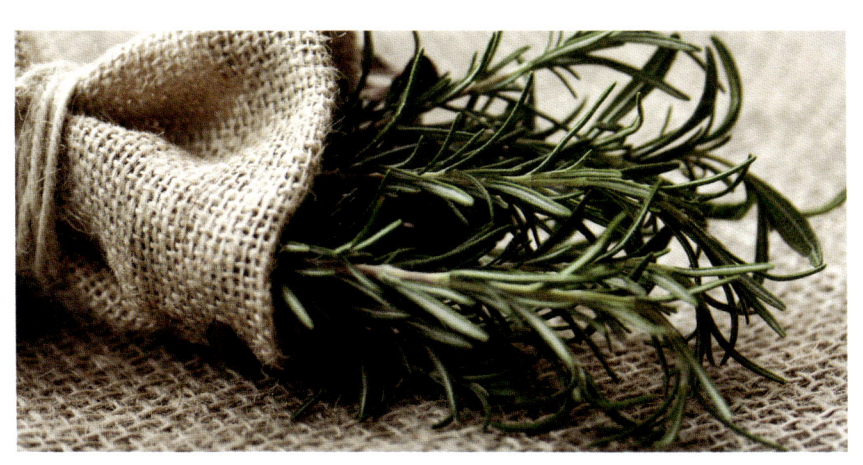

Rosemary, found in a detoxification blend

VAGINITIS

Vaginitis, an infection or inflammation of the vagina, is most common in developing puppies and in overweight adult dogs (See Urinary Conditions and Nutrition). Vaginitis may result from bacterial, viral or fungal infections. Signs of vaginitis include excessive licking of the genital area, increased frequency of urinations, difficulty housebreaking and vaginal discharge.

Clean your dog's vaginal area daily with Gentle Cleanser. Apply Copaiba, Myrrh and Lavender followed with Healing Spray to support the immune system and decrease inflammation and irritation. Diffuse Protective Blend and Frankincense. Feed your pet a high quality diet and supplement with Omega-3 and probiotics.

If signs of vaginitis persist for more than 2–3 days, contact your veterinarian.

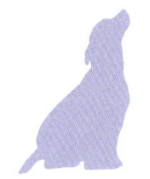

FOR DOGS

Clean your dog's vaginal area 2–4 times daily with Gentle Cleanser.

Apply 1 drop each Copaiba, Myrrh and Lavender in 2 tsp. carrier oil twice daily.

Apply Healing Spray twice daily.

Diffuse Protective Blend or Frankincense for at least 20–30 minutes 2–3 times daily.

Feed your pet a high quality diet and supplement with Omega-3 and probiotics.

If signs of vaginitis persist for more than 2–3 days, contact your veterinarian.

Healing Spray/Healing Oil Blend

Ingredients
5 drops Frankincense Essential Oil
5 drops Geranium Essential Oil
5 drops Lavender Essential Oil
5 drops Helichrysum Essential Oil
5 drops Myrrh Essential Oil
4 oz. water or Aloe Vera Juice for the spray
　　OR
3–4 tsp. carrier oil such as Fractionated Coconut Oil
For dogs only: *If no relief is noted in 24 hours, add 5 drops of Arborvitae to the Healing Spray and Healing Oil Blend.*
4 oz. Glass or Plastic Spray Bottle*
Instructions
Add essential oils to glass or plastic spray bottle. Top with water, Aloe Vera Juice or Carrier Oil. Shake the bottle well before use.

Gentle Cleanser

Ingredients
4 oz. Castile soap or unscented natural foaming soap
2 drops Roman Chamomile Essential Oil
2 drops Lavender Essential Oil
Glass or Plastic Container*
Instructions
Add essential oils to glass or plastic container. Top with soap. Shake the bottle well before use. Lather and rinse well.

VESTIBULAR DISEASE (VESTIBULITIS)

The vestibular system, located in the inner ear, middle ear and brain, is responsible for maintaining normal balance and direction. Vestibulitis, also called old dog vestibular syndrome or canine idiopathic vestibular syndrome, occurs most commonly in older dogs. Vestiubular disease affects cats of any age and cats who are deaf are at higher risk. Siamese and Burmese cat breeds may develop inherited or congenital vestibulitis.

Vestibular disease often develops suddenly and with no known cause. When no cause is determined, the condition is called idiopathic. In other cases, vestibulitis may be associated with ear infections, trauma or injury, certain medications, tumors or hypothyroidism (See Ear Infections, Hypothyroidism, Trauma).

Signs of vestibulitis include dizziness, incoordination, a head tilt to one side, walking in circles, stumbling, falling over, irregular darting eye movements (nystagmus) and vomiting (See Diarrhea and Vomiting).

Vestibular disease is diagnosed with a thorough medical history, physical examination and testing. Signs are most pronounced upon onset of illness and for the first 24–48 hours. Signs generally improve over 7–10 days with full recovery in 2–3 weeks. Rarely, an affected dog may suffer lifelong wobbling or a head tilt.
Treatment may be directed at the cause, if found. For example, attending to an ear infection. In most cases, though, the pets are treated with medication to reduce nausea, vomiting and motion sickness. Pets may need assistance eating and drinking while their sense of balance and direction is altered. Cats may have trouble getting in and out of the litter box safely and easily. In severe cases, the pets may need to be hospitalized and supported until they regain safe, normal equilibrium and mobility. Essential oils can speed recovery and help your pet to return to normal life. Using essential

Ailments, Conditions, and Other Issues

oils such as Cardamom and Digestive Blend help to relieve nausea, vomiting and motion sickness. Grounding Blend is a combination of tree oils which strengthen the connection to the body and to the earth promoting stability and balance. Frankincense supports brain health, regeneration of cells and is useful in trauma and insults to the nervous system. Copaiba is a powerful anti-inflammatory. For dogs and cats, apply Frankincense, Copaiba, Lavender, Melissa, Grounding Blend and Digestive Blend twice daily or more if needed. Diffusing essential oils for your pet with vestibulitis is particularly effective to expose your pet to these oils for a prolonged period of time. We suggest diffusing Grounding Blend, Restful Blend and Frankincense twice daily or more if needed.

To maintain good overall health, feed a high quality diet supplemented with Omega-3 and probiotics.

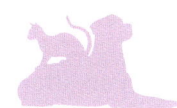

FOR DOGS & CATS

Apply 1 drop each Frankincense, Copaiba, Lavender, Melissa, Grounding Blend and Digestive Blend in 2 tsp. carrier oil (4 tsp. carrier for cats) twice daily or more if needed.

Diffuse a combination of Grounding Blend, Restful Blend and Frankincense for 20–30 minutes 2–3 times daily or more if needed.

Feed a high quality diet supplemented with Omega-3 and probiotics.

WORMS (INTESTINAL PARASITES)

Nearly all puppies and kittens are born with intestinal parasites, which they get from their mother. The parasites are transmitted during pregnancy and nursing. Pets may also become infected with intestinal parasites at any time throughout their lives and via a number of routes. Parasites may be transferred to your pet if they visit an area which is populated with stray animals or rodents that deposit worms wherever they roam. Dogs who frequent dog parks or day care facilities where dogs may congregate or play together are highly susceptible. In addition, worms may even enter our homes on our shoes or from bags or boxes that have been placed on the ground and then brought into our homes. Parasites like intestinal tapeworms are transmitted by fleas (See Fleas, Ticks, and Mosquitoes).

Pet owners may notice worms in the feces when they clean up after their pets. In some cases, parasites will not be visible with the naked eye. Pets infected with parasites may or may not develop diarrhea (See Diarrhea and Vomiting). See your veterinarian for physical exam and diagnostic testing if worms or diarrhea are present. Intestinal parasites may be transmitted to people, so we suggest your pet undergo routine parasite testing.

Responsible pet owners should clean up after their dogs and properly dispose of waste to decrease transmission. Be particularly cautious when cleaning up after your pet(s). as many types of intestinal worms and parasites are also contagious to people. Children are at a higher risk than adults, since they are not as conscientious about cleanliness. Protect yourself and your family by practicing good hygiene. Wash your hands after cleaning up messes, cleaning the litter box or picking up after your pet, prior to cooking, preparing food or eating. Keep children away from the litter box and other dirty areas. In addition, we suggest using a Natural Hand Sanitizer or Protective Blend Sanitizing Mist.

Ailments, Conditions, and Other Issues

Essential oils will complement traditional therapies and support your pet's immune system. As always, feed your pet a high quality diet and supplement with Omega-3 and probiotics.

For dogs, apply Digestive Blend, Arborvitae, Copaiba, Lemongrass (not recommended for puppies, use Lavender instead) and Myrrh daily. Diffuse Protective Blend or Frankincense alternating oils if you wish to support the immune system. For cats, apply Digestive Blend, Arborvitae, Copaiba, Lemongrass (not recommended for kittens, use Lavender) and Myrrh daily. Diffuse Protective Blend or Frankincense alternating oils if you wish to support the immune system. Add Digestive Blend or Myrrh and Lavender to the Litter Box (See Recipes: Litter Box Power).

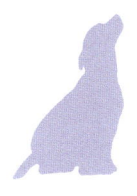

FOR DOGS

Apply 1 drop each Digestive Blend, Arborvitae, Copaiba, Lemongrass (not recommended for puppies, use Lavender) and Myrrh diluted in 2 tsp. carrier oil twice daily.

Diffuse Protective Blend or Frankincense for 20–30 minutes 2–3 times daily.

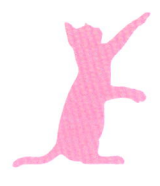

FOR CATS

Apply 1 drop each Digestive Blend, Arborvitae, Copaiba, Lemongrass (not recommended for kittens, use Lavender) and Myrrh diluted in 4 tsp. carrier oil twice daily.

Diffuse Protective Blend or Frankincense for 20–30 minutes 2–3 times daily.

Add Digestive Blend or Myrrh and Lavender to the Litter Box (See Recipes: Litter Box Power).

Natural Hand Sanitizer

Ingredients
5 Tbsp. Aloe Vera Gel
4 Tbsp. water
1/4 tsp. Vitamin E oil
8–10 drops of Protective Essential Oil Blend
Glass or Plastic Container*

Instructions
Add essential oil to an empty glass or plastic container. Add aloe vera gel, water and vitamin E oil. Whisk together all of the ingredients and place in a squeeze bottle for use on the go.

"There's no need for a piece of sculpture in a home that has a cat."

-Wesley Bates

Ailments, Conditions, and Other Issues

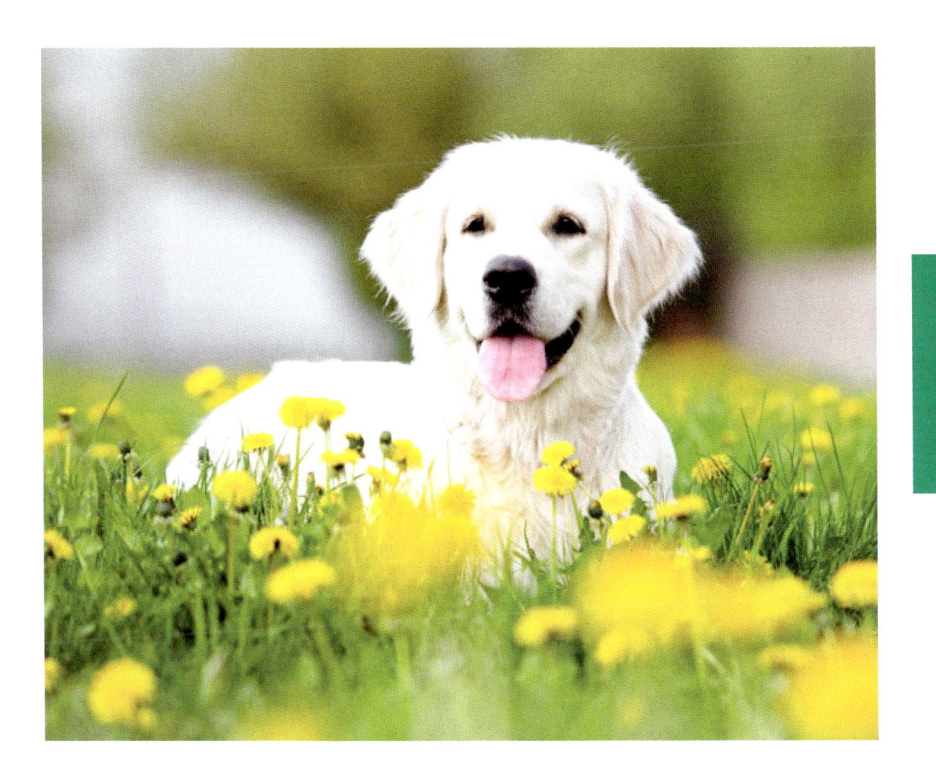

COMMONLY RECOMMENDED ESSENTIAL OILS

Arborvitae means "tree of life" in Latin, and this tree can live for hundreds of years. The Arborvitae, or Western Red Cedar, is native to North America and chemically contains a unique concentration of tropolones, a group of chemical compounds which are highly antiseptic. Although this oil is powerful, it is extremely gentle. Arborvitae is known for its strong insect repellent qualities. This woods aroma provides a peaceful and relaxed sensation (found in Outdoor Blend).

Basil is sometimes known as the royal herb, as the origin of the name comes from the Greek word for king. Historically, Basil was used to help promote feelings of courage and strength. As a natural anti-inflammatory, antiviral, antibiotic and diuretic, basil has been used in traditional Indian medicine practices for centuries. Basil essential oil is also a good option for reducing itching and the pain from bites and stings from bees, insects, and snakes (found in Centering Blend, Massage Blend).

Bergamot, historically was used for fevers and digestive tract problems. It is antibacterial and an antiseptic and has been shown to be effective in treating urinary tract infections. Bergamot is excellent for skin care, and like many citrus oils is calming and therefore helpful with anxiety and depression. It is uplifting and energizing (found in Women's Perfume Blend).

Cardamom, a member of the ginger family is known as the "Queen of Spices" in the cooking world. Used by many cultures worldwide to flavor food and promote healthy digestion. Cardamom contains high amounts of linalool and 1,8-cineole which contributes to Cardamom oil's ability to promote clear airways, easeful breathing, and tranquility. Cardamom is not only calming emotionally but also physically, being useful for digestive upset, constipation, diarrhea and respiratory conditions (found in Respiratory Blend).

Cedarwood is useful for respiratory conditions, skin issues, as well as kidney and urinary tract problems. Cedarwood is high in a natural chemical called cedrol. Cedrol has been found to enhance fibroblast growth in the skin so it is very good for skin recovery. Cedarwood promotes restfulness, feelings of calmness and relaxation (found in Outdoor Blend).

Chamomile (Roman) is an essential oil that has been used for centuries. Roman Chamomile has a broad range of applications including, allergies, burns, diarrhea, nausea, psoriasis, sprains, fever, earaches, teething, and stomach aches. It is beneficial for many skin conditions, including burns, cuts abrasions and insect bites. Roman Chamomile has calming and relaxing properties. It can help with anxiety, depression, insomnia, and restlessness (found in Focus Blend, Restful Blend).

Cobaiba essential oil is distilled from the oleo-resin of the Copaiba balsam tree that grows in the Amazon forests of Brazil and has been utilized since the 16th century for health purposes. Rich in Beta-caryophyllene and other sesquiterpenes, which act synergistically so as to have a therapeutic effect on many different body systems, Copaiba essential oil supports the health of the nervous, cardiovascular, immune, digestive, musculoskeletal and respiratory systems. It is a powerful antioxidant and is one of the most anti-inflammatory chemicals found in nature. Copaiba also offers anti-tumoral properties and helps to promote healthy skin.

Cypress is particularly beneficial for improving circulation and lymphatic drainage. Cypress may be useful for strengthening blood capillary walls, the circulatory system, edema, lung circulation, and liver disorders. Cypress is helpful at healing wounds quickly. Emotionally Cypress assists in dealing with feelings of loss, grief and promoting confidence (found in Massage Blend).

Eucalyptus is known for respiratory support and is useful for allergies, asthma, colds, and fevers. It not only helps relieve the symptoms but also has antibacterial and antiviral properties. Eucalyptol, or 1,8-cineole, which accounts for 70–90 percent of the contents of Eucalyptus, has antioxidant, anti-inflammatory and pain-relieving properties. It is also helpful to repel pests (found in Protective Blend, Outdoor Blend, and Respiratory Blend).

Frankincense is a wondrous oil. It is beneficial for numerous conditions and body systems. Use Frankincense for neurologic disorders, autoimmune disorders, respiratory illness, depression, and to restore life force. Frankincense has been extensively studied for it's anti-tumoral properties. Frankincense reduces heart rate and high blood pressure and is calming and centering. When in doubt, use Frankincense (found in Anti-aging Blend, Cellular Complex Blend, Focus Blend, and Grounding Blend).

Geranium is used heavily in the perfume and cosmetic industry. For this reason, it is important to be assured of the purity and quality of the essential oil that you are using, since there are lower quality products easily available. Geranium aids hormonal balance, , is antiseptic and aids in treatment of skin and ear infections and reduces bruising. . Geranium oil helps repair and maintain healthy skin as it inhibits the inflammatory responses in the skin. Geranium has been found to be a useful bug repellent and particularly effective against ticks (found in Detoxification Blend).

Grapefruit is refreshing and uplifting, helps to resolve anger and irritability. It supports lymphatic drainage, improves digestion and relieves muscle fatigue. Grapefruit is high in a compound called d-limonene, which is beneficial in cancer prevention and support (found in Massage Blend).

Helichrysum contains natural chemicals that renew and calm tissue. It has antifungal and antimicrobial properties and is helpful for respiratory illnesses, skin conditions, painfulness and neurologic conditions. Specifically, it is useful for skin irritations, bruising, sprains and joint or arthritic pain. It has very strong anti-inflammatory properties and has been known to aid in blood circulation and hypertension. Helichrysum is also beneficial in the detoxification and stimulation of liver cell function Emotionally is healing to bruised emotions, resentment and anger (found in Anti-aging Blend).

Lavender is a very versatile oil known for its calming properties. Lavender is an adaptogen, meaning it can assist the body when adapting to stress or imbalances. It is a natural antihistamine, antiviral, and helpful for dry skin, burns, bruises, cuts, and woundsLavender reduces feelings of fear and hiding and instills a sense of peace. (found in Anti-aging Blend, Comforting Blend and Restful Blend).

Lemon is a powerful immune stimulant. Lemon is cleansing to the kidneys and the liver and is antibacterial and antifungal. Lemon is useful to sharpen focus and reduce confusion. It is uplifting, energizing, and is high in a compound called d-limonene, which is beneficial in cancer prevention and support (found in Cleansing Blend and Respiratory Blend).

Lemongrass (hot oil) is beneficial for thyroid conditions and for hormonal balance. It is a very effective pain reliever, kills fungal and viral infections and is antitumoral. In addition, Lemongrass helps to clear the mind, ground the body and relieve anxiety. It is also an effective insect repellent (found in Cellular Complex Blend).

Magnolia blossoms must be picked by hand early in the morning or late in the evening in order to extract the essential oil. Magnolia essential oil is high in linalool which is very soothing and relaxing to the emotions. Magnolia is supportive in times of anxiety, grief, depression, anger and loneliness.

Marjoram, to the Greeks and Romans, was a symbol of happiness. It is a powerful analgesic and helps in pain management and is helpful for sore muscle and joints. Marjoram can have positive effects on the nervous, immune, and cardiovascular systems improving blood flow and lowering blood pressure. Marjoram, promotes healthy joint function, skin and hair health, and proper immune system function. Marjoram helps to instill feelings of trust and connection especially after loss or harsh life experiences (found in Centering Blend, Massage Blend).

Melaleuca is a powerful antiseptic oil. Use Melaleuca to help kill airborne viruses, bacteria and fungal infections and is beneficial for treating wounds and skin conditions. Melaleuca, also known as Tea Tree oil, is well known for it's cleansing and soothing properties fortifying the lungs and offering feelings of confidence and security. We recommend Melaleuca to be used only in difficult and resistant cases and guided by your veterinarian (found in Cleansing Blend and Respiratory Blend).

Myrrh stimulates the immune system and blood circulation. Thus, Myrrh helps to relieve pain, subdue swelling and promote tissue regeneration. It is a potent antimicrobial, analgesic, useful in thyroid conditions, cancer, diabetes, digestive issues and wounds. Historically, Myrrh is considered the mother oil, has nurturing characteristics and promotes feelings of security, love and trust (found in Anti-aging Blend).

Oregano (hot oil) is a powerful anti-inflammatory and is nature's antibiotic, effective against MRSA and other infectious agents. Oregano is powerful against viruses, fungal organisms, bacteria, parasites and warts. We recommend Oregano to be used only under the guidance of your veterinarian.

Peppermint is soothing for painful conditions, indigestion, vomiting, diarrhea, congestion, fever, and allergies. It is beneficial in dental care due to its antiseptic properties and helps to clear the respiratory tract and ease breathing. Also, found to improve concentration, energy and mental sharpness (found in Digestive Blend, Massage Blend, and Respiratory Blend).

Pink Pepper brings with it a unique blend of constituents and a chemical profile that bears several health-supporting benefits. What makes the chemistry of Pink Pepper so unique is that it includes a very high concentration of alpha-phellandrene which has a profound effect on immune cells. This makes Pink Pepper excellent at promoting the body's natural healing process, ease discomfort, and support normal inflammatory function.

Rose is known as the queen of flowers and over 12,000 rose blossoms are required to make one 5 ml bottle of Rose essential oil. Rose holds the highest vibration of any oil and is a wonderful healer of the heart. Thus, it is comforting in times of depression and loss. Rose is well recognized for its emotional benefits but has powerful effects on the brain and nervous system, is antibacterial and antitumoral (found in Anti-Aging Blend, Comforting Blend, and Women's Perfume Blend).

Sandalwood promotes a feeling of calm and is useful in depression and anxiety. Sandalwood contains alpha-santalol, which helps protect against skin cancer. It balances moisture in the skin and is healing for dry skin conditions and scars (found in Anti-aging Blend).

Thyme was given to knights and warriors before they went into battle by ladies as it was thought to impart courage to its bearer. Thyme is a potent antibacterial and antiviral and helps to clear congestion in the respiratory system. Thyme is cleansing and purifying and helps to promote healthy cellular replication and function. We recommend Thyme only be used with the guidance of your veterinarian (found in Detoxification Blend).

Turmeric or "Sacred Earth" in Latin is best known for a variety of benefits. Turmeric contains two classes of chemicals, curcuminoids and turmerones, that have a powerful impact on the body. Curcuminoids are large, water-soluble molecules whose absorption is improved by Turmeric essential oil. Tumerones are tiny, fat-soluble molecules that readily absorb into the bloodstream and are found in Turmeric oil. The use of Turmeric oil has a profound effect on regulating inflammation and on cellular health. It is advantageous for neurological conditions, autoimmune disorders, joint pain, and is highly antiseptic (found in Polyphenol Complex).

Vetiver is a member of the grass family, and the fragrance is earthy and strong. Unlike other grasses, the root system of Vetiver grows down, making it ideal for helping prevent erosion and providing soil stabilization. Vetiver is very calming, grounding, centering and focusing. Vetiver is helpful for anxiety, insecurity, restlessness, and insomnia (found in Focus Blend, Women's Perfume Blend). Wild Orange has a very powerful sweet scent and is useful for purifying the air and eliminating odors. The antibacterial properties in wild orange oil make it an excellent natural cleaning product (found in Cellular Complex Blend, Protective Blend and Outdoor Blend).

Ylang Ylang also helps to regulate blood pressure and hormones. Historically, it was used for skin treatments, insect bites, hair loss, digestive issues and for the respiratory system. Ylang Ylang is useful as an antidepressant, promoting emotional balance, feelings of joy and playfulness(found in Focus Blend, Joyful Blend, Outdoor Blend, Restful Blend, and Women's Perfume Blend).

*Cassia and Black Pepper are hot oils and are only recommended in this book for deterring pets from chewing and destructive behavior. These oils have many uses but we do not recommend their use in pets.

Recipes

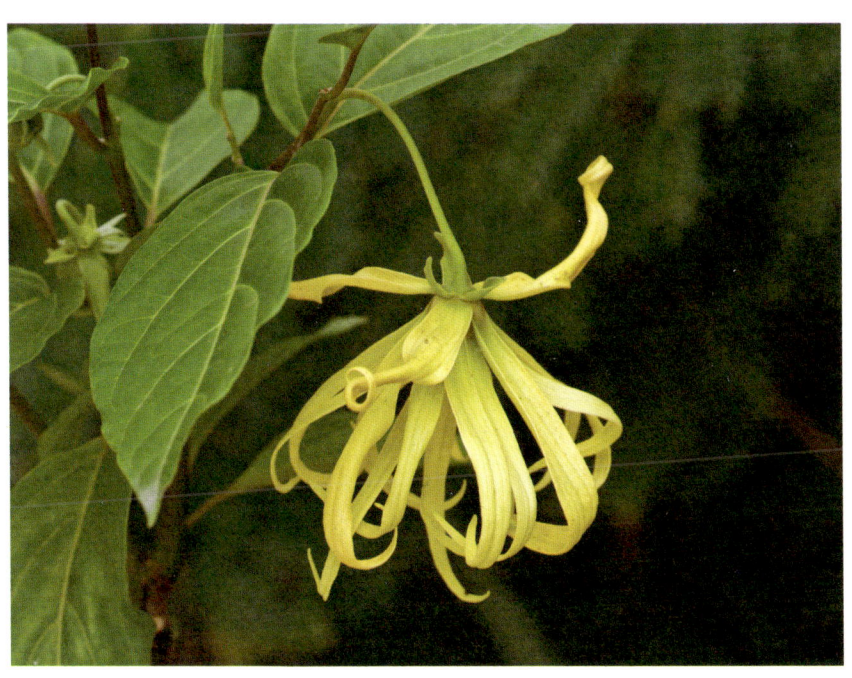

Ylang Ylang

SpOil Your Pet

RECIPES

Antiseptic Shampoo
10 oz. Water
2 oz. Aloe Vera
1 Tbsp. Castile soap
2 drops Myrrh Essential Oil
2 drops Lavender Essential Oil
2 drops Geranium Essential Oil
2 drops Cleansing Essential Oil Blend
Glass or Plastic Bottle*

Add essential oils to an empty bottle. Add castile soap, aloe vera juice and water. Shake the bottle well before use. Lather and rinse well.

Chew Deterrent Spray with Essential Oils
5–6 drops of Cassia Essential Oil
or Black Pepper Essential Oil
or Citrus Essential Oil
4 oz. Water
Glass or Plastic Spray Bottle*

Add essential oils to a 4 oz. glass or plastic spray bottle and fill with water. Shake the bottle well before use. Test the spray on a hidden area of your furniture (or other object which your puppy/dog likes to chew) to ensure it will not stain or mark the item. Spray generously and reapply as the smell wears off. If the spray does not seem to be working well, add more of the essential oil or prepare the Chew Deterrent Spray with a different hot essential oil.

Flea & Tick Repellent Shampoo or Spray
8 oz. Natural Shampoo Base or Water
4 drops Clary Sage Essential Oil
2 drops Cleansing Essential Oil Blend
5 drops Repellant Essential Oil Blend
8 drops Peppermint Essential Oil

4 drops Lemon Essential Oil
2 drops Geranium Essential Oil
2 drops Eucalyptus Essential Oil
3 drops Lavender Essential Oil
2 drops Myrrh Essential Oil
2 drops Thyme Essential Oil
Glass or Plastic Bottle*

Add essential oils to an empty glass or plastic bottle. Top with water. Shake the bottle well before use. Spray your pet, bedding and yourself!

Gentle Cleanser

4 oz. Castile soap or unscented natural foaming soap
2 drops Roman Chamomile Essential Oil
2 drops Lavender Essential Oil
Glass or Plastic Container*

Add essential oils to glass or plastic container. Top with soap. Shake the bottle well before use. Lather and rinse well.

Healing Salve

8 oz. Cold-Pressed Organic Coconut Oil
1 oz. Beeswax
2 drops Vitamin E (optional)
10 drops Lavender Essential Oil
5 drops Myrrh Essential Oil
3 drops Helichrysum Essential Oil
Glass Jars , Tin Containers or Plastic Bottle *

Place the coconut oil and beeswax over a double–boiler, and gently warm over low heat until the beeswax melts. Remove from heat and add the essential oils and Vitamin E oil, (if using). Quickly pour the mixture into glass jars, tins, or plastic containers and allow to cool completely. Store salve in a cool location where it will not re-melt and re-solidify. When stored correctly, salve will last for 1–3 years. Yields 8 oz.

Healing Spray/Healing Oil Blend

5 drops Frankincense Essential Oil
5 drops Geranium Essential Oil
5 drops Lavender Essential Oil
5 drops Helichrysum Essential Oil
5 drops Myrrh Essential Oil
4 oz. water or Aloe Vera Juice for the spray
　　OR
3–4 tsp. carrier oil such as Fractionated Coconut Oil
For dogs only: If no relief is noted in 24 hours, add 5 drops of Arborvitae to the Healing Spray and Healing Oil Blend.
4 oz. Glass or Plastic Spray Bottle*
Add essential oils to glass or plastic spray bottle. Top with water, Aloe Vera Juice or Carrier Oil. Shake the bottle well before use.

Homemade Doggie Toothpaste

1 Tbsp. Baking Soda
1 Tbsp. Bentonite Clay
1 Tbsp. Solid Organic Coconut Oil
1 drop Peppermint Essential Oil
1 drop Myrrh Essential Oil
Glass or Plastic Container*
Add the coconut oil to a glass bowl and whisk well. Add the baking soda and bentonite clay to the coconut oil and mix thoroughly. Add essential oils to this mixture. Store in a glass or plastic container in a cool place. Makes a 1 month supply if used daily.

Homemade Flea Collar

5 drops Eucalyptus Essential Oil
5 drops Geranium Essential oil
5 drops Thyme Essential Oil
5 drops Lemongrass Essential Oil
5 drops Repellant Essential Oil Blend
4 oz. distilled water
Glass or Plastic Container*
For puppies younger than 4 months or for dogs weighing less than 15 pounds,

use 2 drops of each recommended essential oil in 8 oz. of distilled water.
For cats, use 1 drop each Arborvitae, Geranium, Thyme, Lemongrass, and Repellant Blend in 8 oz. of distilled water.

Mix distilled water with the essential oils in a glass or plastic container. Soak a nylon/cloth collar in the solution for 20 minutes. Remove collar and allow it to dry thoroughly before placing it on your pet. Re-soak the collar every two weeks or more frequently as needed.

Litter Box Power
2–3 drops Essentail Oils
1 Cup Baking Soda
Glass Jar or Plastic Container*

Add 2–3 drops of the chosen essential oil(s) to 1 cup of baking soda. Allow the mixture to rest overnight in a glass jar. Add 1 Tbsp. of the mixture of essential oil and baking soda recipe to the litter box daily.

Some of Our Favorite Combinations:

For Calming: Add 1 drop each Lavender, Copaiba and Roman Chamomile Essential Oils

For Digestive Issues: Add 1 drop each Digestive Blend, Myrrh and Lavender Essential Oils

For Kidney and Bladder Issues: Add 1 drop each Juniper Berry and Ylang Ylang or Lavender Essential Oils

For Overall Health: Add 1 drop each Frankincense, Copaiba, and Lavender Essential Oils

For Odor Control: Add 2 drops Cleansing Blend or Rosemary Essential Oils

For Pain: Add 1 drop each Lavender, Frankincense, and Copaiba Essential Oils

Natural Ear Cleaner

1 oz. Witch Hazel
1 oz. Apple Cider Vinegar
Glass or Plastic Bowl

Combine witch hazel and apple cider vinegar in a a glass or plastic bowl. Generously apply 1–3 tsp. of natural ear cleaner and massage the ear canal. Either pour the cleaner into the ear canal and massage, or saturate a cotton ball, place it at the top of the ear canal, and massage the ear to release the fluid. Remove the cotton ball. Proceed with wiping out the ear canal with dry cotton balls. (The cotton ball method is useful for cats.)

Natural Flea Bomb

10 drops Black Pepper Essential Oil
10 drops Oregano Essential Oil
10 drops Orange Essential Oil
10 drops Peppermint Essential Oil
10 drops Cleansing Essential Oil Blend (to be used after "flea bombing" the house)

Add the essential oils to a water diffuser or in an empty bottle for a nebulizer diffuser. Open all the interior doors in your home and place the diffuser in the most central location possible. If there is a heavy infestation in more than one room you will need to treat each room individually. Turn your diffuser on to maximum output and use a continuous diffusion for 2–3 hours. Leave your home during this time and take your pets with you if possible. If you are not able to take your pets try to keep them in a separate room away from the diffuser. Upon returning home, open all the windows in your home. Diffuse Cleansing Blend for another 1–2 hours.

Now it is time to vacuum everywhere! Move furniture and vacuum behind it and under it. Vacuum the furniture, too. Empty the vacuum when you are finished, and discard any contents outside of your home.

Recipes

Natural Hand Sanitizer
5 Tbsp. Aloe Vera Gel
4 Tbsp. water
1/4 tsp. Vitamin E oil
8–10 drops of Protective Essential Oil Blend
Glass or Plastic Container*
Add essential oil to an empty glass or plastic container. Add aloe vera gel, water and vitamin E oil. Whisk together all of the ingredients and place in a squeeze bottle for use on the go.

Natural Spider-Stay-Away-Spray
16 oz. warm water
1 Tbsp. liquid dish soap
1 Tbsp. white vinegar (optional)
5–7 drops Peppermint Essential Oil
5–7 drops Melaleuca Essential Oil
5–7 drops Lavender Essential Oil
Glass or Plastic Spray Bottle*
Put 5–7 drops of each essential oil in an empty glass or plastic spray bottle and fill mostly to the top with warm water. Add 1 tablespoon of natural dish soap, replace the top. Shake the bottle well before use. Spray the corners of window frames, along door cracks, or in dark, dingy places spiders may be hiding out. You may also add a teaspoon of white vinegar to the mixture, but keep in mind that vinegar may affect some fabrics and surfaces.

Pet Powder
1 Cup Corn Starch
5 drops Lavender Essential Oil
5 drops Geranium Essential Oil
4 drops Eucalyptus Essential Oil
Glass or Plastic Container*
Add baking soda to a glass or plastic container. Add essential oils. Mix well, and keep in a small mason jar with several holes in the top. Sprinkle a small amount on your dog and brush him or her. He or she will not only smell great, but repels ticks and other pests.

Soothing Skin Shampoo

3 oz. Castile soap (available at many health and bulk food stores)
2 oz. Organic Unpasteurized, Unfiltered Apple Cider Vinegar
1 oz. Vegetable Glycerin
2 oz. Distilled water
3 drops Lavender Essential Oil
3 drops Roman Chamomile Essential Oil
3 drops Myrrh Essential Oil
Optional: *add 1 tsp. Ground Oatmeal*
Glass or Plastic Bottle*
Add essential oils to an empty glass or plastic bottle. Add ground oatmeal (if using). Add the apple cider vinegar, vegetable glycerin, and water to the bottle containing essential oils and oatmeal. Add the castile soap. Shake the bottle well before use.

Sunburn/Skin Healing Spray

1 oz. Aloe Vera Juice
2–4 drops Lavender Essential Oil
1 drop Helichrysum Essential Oil
4 oz. Glass or Plastic Spray Bottle*
Place all ingredients in a glass or plastic spray bottle. Shake the bottle well before use. Spray the affected area, taking caution to avoid your pet's eyes. You may spray some of the mixture into your hands and carefully apply to your pet's face, head and muzzle.

Note: Try to purchase the best quality aloe vera possible. Aloe vera products that contain synthetics will dry the skin and will not help the skin to heal from a sunburn or skin condition.

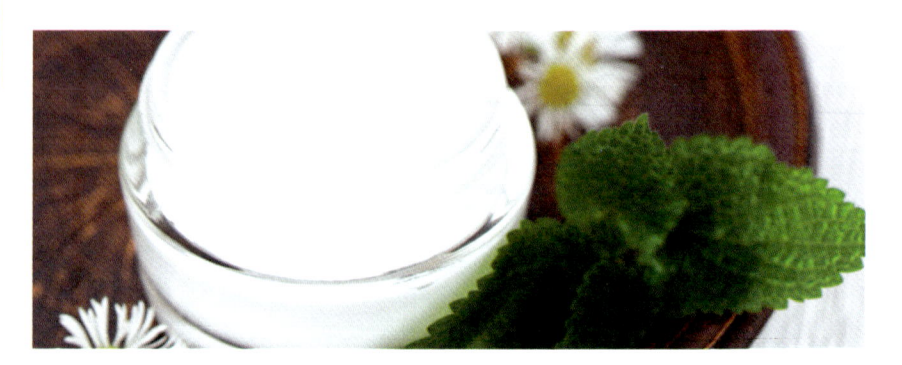

Recipes

Urine Odor Eliminating Spray

5 oz. Hydrogen Peroxide
1 tsp. Vinegar
1 tsp. Baking Soda
3 drops Wild Orange Essential Oil
Glass or plastic spray bottle*

Add the essential oil to the empty bottle. Add the baking soda followed by the vinegar and hydrogen peroxide. Shake the bottle well before use. Now simply spray the affected area generously with the solution and allow to completely dry. It will become powder-like once the formula dries. Once it dries, vacuum up the powder.
If the smell remains, spray and vacuum again and follow with the powder described below.

Urine Odor Eliminating Powder

1 cup Baking Soda
3 drops Lemon Essential Oil
3 drops Rosemary Essential Oil
Glass or Plastic Container*

Add essential oils to the baking soda. Place into a glass or plastic container and shake until well combined.
Sprinkle the powder on the dry affected area and leave on for several hours or overnight and vacuum again.

*__Note:__ Glass containers are preferred for all recipes, but BPA-free plastic containers can work as a substitute if needed when using heavily-diluted essential oils.

REFERENCES

Bae GS, Park KC, Choi SB, et al. Protective effects of alpha-pinene in mice with cerulein-induced acute pancreatitis. Life Sci. 2012;91(17–18):866–871.

Bell KL. (2002)vHolistic Aromatherapy for Animals: A Comprehensive Guide to the Use of Essential Oils & Hydrosols with Animals, Findhorn Press, Forres Scotland, UK

Center for Disease Control, Tick Borne Diseases, NIOSH Fast Facts Card: Protecting Yourself from Ticks and Mosquitoes, 2010-119

Chen Y, Zhou C, Ge Z, et al. Composition and potential anticancer activities of essential oils obtained from myrrh and frankincense. Oncol Lett. 2013;6(4):1140-1146.

Chin KB, Cordell B. The effect of tea tree oil (Melaleuca alternifolia) on wound healing using a dressing model. J Altern Complement Med. 2013;19(12):942-945.

Cornell Feline Health Center, Feline Immunodeficiency Virus 2019

Cornell Feline Health Center, Feline Leukemia Virus 2016

Crowell PL, Gould MN. Chemoprevention and therapy of cancer by d-limonene. Crit Rev. Oncog. 5 (1):1-22, 1994.

de Sousa AA, Soares PM, de Almeida AN, et al. Antispasmodic effect of Mentha piperita essential oil on tracheal smooth muscle of rats. J Ethnopharmacol. 2010;130(2):422-436.

Douillard, J. Detox Your Brain & Guts with Fish Oils 2018

References

Elegbede JA, Elson CE, Qureshi A, et al. Inhibition of DMBA induced mammary cancer by the monoterpene d-limonene. Carcinogenesis 5 (5):661-664, 1984

Elson CE, Maltzman T H, Boston JL, et al. Anti-carcinogenic activity of d-limonene during the initiation and promotion/progression stages of DMBA-induced rat mammary carcinogenesis. Carcinogenesis 9 (2):331-332, 1988.

Emotions and Essential Oils: A Reference for Emotional Healing 7th Edition, 2019.

Fan AY, Lao L, Zhang RX, et al. Effects of an acetone extract of Boswellia carterii Birdw. (Burseraceae) gum resin on adjuvant-induced arthritis in lewis rats. J Ethnopharmacol. 2005;101(1-3):104-109.

Feldman, E. Cushing's Disease in Dogs American College of Veterinary Internal Medicine, 2014

Frank MB, Yang Q, Osban J, et al. Frankincense oil derived from Boswellia carteri induces tumor cell specific cytotoxicity. BMC Complement Altern Med. 2009 Mar 18;9:6

Gilani AH, Jabeen Q, Khan AU, Shah AJ. Gut modulatory, blood pressure lowering, diuretic and sedative activities of cardamom. J Ethnopharmacol. 2008 Feb 12;115(3):463-72.

Graham L, Wells, DL, Hepper PG. The influence of olfactory stimulation on the behaviour of dogs housed in a rescue shelter. Appl Anim Behav Sci. 2005;91(1-2):143-153.

Haag JD, Lindstrom MJ, Gould MN. Limonene-induced regression of mammary carcinomas. Cancer Res. 52 (14):4021-4026, 1992.

Hancianu M, Cioanca O, Mihasan M, et al. Neuroprotective effects of inhaled lavender oil on scopolamine-induced dementia via anti-oxidative activities in rats. Phytomedicine. 2013;20(5):446-452.

Haque M, Coury DL. Topical Sandalwood Oil for Common Warts. Clin Pediatr 2018: 57(1):93-95.

Holmes C, Hopkins V, Hensford C, et al. Lavender oil as a treatment for agitated behaviour in severe dementia: a placebo controlled study. International Journal of Geriatric Psychiatry. 2002;17:305-308.

Homburger, F, Treger, A, Boger, E. Inhibition of Murine Subcutaneous and Intravenous Benzo(rst) Pentaphene. Carcinogenesis by Sweet Orange Oils and D-Limonene. Oncology, 25(1):1-10, 1971.

Hsu WS, Yen JH, Wang YS. Formulas of components of citronella oil against mosquitoes (Aedes Egypt). J Environ Sci Health B. 2013;48(11):1014-1019.

Hunter, T, Ward E. Snakebite Envenomization, VCA, Veterinary Centers of America 2019

Ishak, WW, Kahloon, M, Fakhry, H. Oxytocin role in enhancing well-being: A literature review [Abstract]. J Affective Disorders 2011; 130(1-2), 1-9.

Jimbo D, Kimura Y, Taniguchi M, et al. Effect of aromatherapy on patients with Alzheimer's disease. Phychogeriatrics. 2009;9(4):173-179.

References

Johannessen B. Nurses experience of aromatherapy use with dementia patients experiencing disturbed sleep patterns. An action research project. Complement Ther Clin Pract. 2013;19(4):209-213.

Kannappan S, Jayaraman T, Rajasekar P, et al. Cinnamon bark extract improves glucose metabolism and lipid profile in the fructose-fed rat. Singapore Med J. 2006;47(10):858-863.

Kim HM, Cho SH. Lavender oil inhibits immediate-type allergic reaction in mice and rats. J Pharm Pharmacol. 1999; 51(2):221-226.

Koca Kutlu A, Ceçen D, Gürgen SG, et al. A Comparison Study of Growth Factor Expression following Treatment with Transcutaneous Electrical Nerve Stimulation, Saline Solution, Povidone-Iodine, and Lavender Oil in Wounds Healing. Evid Based Complement Alternat Med. 2013;2013:361832.

Lai TK, Cheung MC, Lo CK, et al. Effectiveness of aroma massage on advanced cancer patients with constipation: a pilot study. Complement Ther Clin Pract. 2011;17(1):37-43.

Lawal HO, Adewuyi GO, Fawehinmi AB. Chemical evaluation of mosquito repellent formulation prepared from the essential oil of plants. J Nat Products. 2013;6:33-37.

Lin PW, Chan WC, Ng BF, et al. Efficacy of aromatherapy (Lavandula angustifolia) as an intervention for agitated behaviours in Chinese older persons with dementia: a cross-over randomized trial. International Journal of Geriatric Psychiatry. 2007 Mar 7.

Lv YX, Zhao SP, Zhang JY, et al. Effect of orange peel essential oil on oxidative stress in AOM animals. Int J Biol Macromol. 2012;50(4):1144-1150.

Martinez K, De Santiago L, Care S, et al. Antibacterial Effects of commercial essential oils on bacteria. J Nat Sci. 2012;1(1):1-3.

Martinez-Velazquez M, Castillo-Herrera GA, Rosario-Cruz R. Acaricidal effect and chemical composition of essential oils extracted from Cuminum cyminum, Pimenta dioica and Ocimum basilicum against the cattle tick Rhipicephalus (Boophilus) microplus (Acari: Ixodidae). Parasitol Res. 2011;108(2):481-487.

McKay DL, Blumberg JB. A review of the bioactivity and potential health benefits of peppermint tea (Mentha piperita L.). Phytother Res. 2006;20(8):619-633.

Mishra A, Bhatti R, Singh A, et al. Ameliorative effect of the cinnamon oil from Cinnamomum zeylanicum upon early stage diabetic nephropathy. Planta Med. 2010;76(5):412-417.

Misner BD. A novel aromatic oil compound inhibits microbial overgrowth on feet: a case study. J Int Soc Sports Nutr. 2007;4:3.

Modern Essentials: The Contemporary Guide to Therapeutic Use of Essential Oils (10th Ed 2018) Orem, UT, AromaTools

Moon SE, Kim HY, Cha JD. Synergistic effect between clove oil and its major compounds and antibiotics against oral bacteria. Arch Oral Biol. 2011;56(9):907-916.

Moore, CJ, Kerman, WS, Wang, BC, Gould, MN, Inhibition of Ras-induced mammary carcinogenesis by limonene. Proc Am Assoc Cancer Res, 32:131, 1991.

References

Morag, N, Essential Oils for Animals: Your complete guide to using aromatherapy for animal health and management. Off The Leash Press. LLC, 2011

Moussaieff A, Shein NA, Tsenter J. Incensole acetate: a novel neuroprotective agent isolated from Boswellia carterii. J Cereb Blood Flow Metab. 2008;28(7):1341-1352.

Mugnaini L, Nardoni S, Pinto L, Pistelli L, et al.In vitro and in vivo anti-fungal activity of some essential oils against feline isolates of Microsporum canis. J Mycol Med. 2012 Jun;22(2):179-84.

Ni X, Suhail MM, Yang Q, Cao A, et al. Frankincense essential oil prepared from hydrodistillation of Boswellia sacra gum resins induces human pancreatic cancer cell death in cultures and in a xenograft murine model. BMC Complement Altern Med. 2012 D;12:253.

Nomicos EY. Myrrh: medical marvel or myth of the Magi? Holist Nurs Pract. 2007;21(6):308-323.

Nostro A, Blanco AR, Cannatelli MA, et al. Susceptibility of methicillin-resistant staphylococci to oregano essential oil, carvacrol and thymol. FEMS Microbiol Lett. Jan;230(2):191-195.

O'Flaherty LA, van Dijk M, Albertyn R, et al. Aromatherapy massage seems to enhance relaxation in children with burns: an observational pilot study. Burns. 2012;38(6):840-845.

Pajer, N. Probiotics for Cats: What are They and How Do They Help? PetMD

Pepeljnjak S, Kosalec I, Kalodera Z, et al. Antimicrobial activity of juniper berry essential oil (Juniperus communis L., Cupressaceae). Acta Pharm. 2005;55(4):417-422.

PetMD Cushing's Disease in Dogs

Picon PD, Picon RV, Costa AF, et al. Randomized clinical trial of a phytotherapic compound containing Pimpinella anisum, Foeniculum vulgare, Sambucus nigra, and Cassia augustifolia for chronic constipation. BMC Complement Altern Med. 2010;10:17(1-9).

Plotnick, A. Can Probiotics Help Your Cat? Cummins School of Veterinary Medicine at Tufts University 2017

Ritter AM, Domiciano TP, Verri WA Jr, Et Al. Antihypernociceptive activity of anethole in experimental inflammatory pain. Inflammopharmacology. 2013;21(2):187-197.

Sala A, Recio M, Giner RM, et al. Anti-inflammatory and antioxidant properties of Helichrysum italicum. J Pharm Pharmacol. 2002;54(3):365-371.

Schnitzler P Essential Oils for the Treatment of Herpes Simplex Virus Infections. Chemotherapy. 2019;64(1):1-7.

Setzer WN. Essential oils and anxiolytic aromatherapy. Nat Prod Commun. 2009;4(9):1305-1316.

Shelton M, (2018) The Animal Desk Reference: Essential Oils for Animals, Howard Lake, MN

References

Shen J, Niijima A, Tanida M, et al. Olfactory stimulation with scent of lavender oil affects autonomic nerves, lipolysis and appetite in rats. Neurosci Lett. 2005;383(1-2):188-193.

Singh D, Kumar TR, Gupt VK, et al. Antimicrobial activity of some promising plant oils, molecules and formulations. Indian J Exp Biol. 2012;50(10):714-717.

Singh, R, Gautam, N, Mishra, A, GuptaIndian, R. Heavy metals and living systems: An overview J Pharmacol. 2011 May-Jun; 43(3): 246–253.

Srivastava JK, Shankar E, Gupta S. Chamomile: A herbal medicine of the past with bright future. Mol Med Rep. 2010;3(6):895-901.

Talpur N, Echard B, Ingram C, et al. Effects of a novel formulation of essential oils on glucose-insulin metabolism in diabetic and hypertensive rats: a pilot study. Diabetes Obes Metab. 2005; 7(2):193-199.

The Natren Blog Could Your Anxious Dog Benefit from Probiotics? 2016

The Essential Life Total Wellness Publishing, LLC, 2018

Thorsell W, Mikiver A, Tunón H. Repelling properties of some plant materials on the tick Ixodes ricinus L. Phytomedicine. 2006;13(1-2):132-134.

Ueno-Iio T, Shibakura M, Yokota K et al. Lavender essential oil inhalation suppresses allergic airway inflammation and mucous cell hyperplasia in a murine model of asthma. Life Sci. 2014

Volhard W, Brown, K. (2000) Holistic Guide for a Healthy Dog (2nd Ed), Hobokre, NJ, Wiley Publishing House

Wallenberg, LW, Coccia, JB. Inhibition of 4-(methylnitrosamino)-1-(3-pyridyl)-1-butanone Carcinogenesis in Mice by D-Limonene and Citrus Fruit Oils. Carcinogenesis, Vol. 12, No. 1, pp. 115-117, 1991

Ward, E, Gollakner, R. Cushing's Disease in Dogs 2017; Life Learn Inc.

Wells DL. Aromatherapy for travel-induced excitement in dogs. J Am Vet Med Assoc. 2006;229(6):964-967.

Woollard AC, Tatham KC, Barker S. The influence of essential oils on the process of wound healing: a review of the current evidence. J Wound Care. 2007;16(6):255-257.

Yabsley, M. Companion Animal Parasite Council (CAPC) Parasite Prevalence Maps 2019

Yavari Kia P, Safajou F, Shahnazi M, Et Al. The effect of lemon inhalation aromatherapy on nausea and vomiting of pregnancy: a double-blinded, randomized, controlled clinical trial. Iran Red Crescent Med J. 2014;16(3):e14360.

References

INDEX

A

Abscess 20, 36, 188, 189, 286
Acid Reflux 24, 286
Acne 103, 286
Addison's Disease 26, 27, 286
Aggressive Behavior 28, 286
Allergies 32, 36, 71, 96, 103, 160, 161, 192, 193, 208, 253, 256, 286
Anal Glands 36, 286
Anorexia 26, 38, 111, 167, 175, 286
Antibacterial 32, 73, 74, 75, 76, 252, 254, 255, 257, 258, 272
Antibiotic 20, 50, 73, 95, 106, 188, 198, 219, 252, 256, 272
Anti-fungal 32, 195, 196, 254, 255, 273
Anti-infectious 32, 150
Anti-inflammatory 32, 95, 119, 150, 247, 252, 253, 254, 256, 274
Antioxidant 31, 48, 59, 63, 64, 180, 206, 212, 253, 254, 274
Antiseptic 8, 22, 33, 74, 77, 78, 195, 196, 197, 198, 199, 200, 252, 254, 256, 258
Anxiety 24, 26, 28, 31, 38, 40, 48, 52, 60, 63, 64, 65, 66, 69, 71, 72, 84, 86, 100, 101, 105, 131, 143, 144, 163, 179, 180, 204, 205, 206, 211, 212, 234, 238, 252, 253, 255, 257, 258, 286
Appetite 20, 27, 38, 39, 59, 71, 83, 87, 89, 105, 108, 121, 139, 173, 188, 219, 275, 286
Arborvitae 21, 51, 192
Arthritis 30, 44, 161, 173, 218, 269, 286
Asthma 192, 275
Autoimmune 47, 150, 286

B

Bartonella 50, 114, 286
Basil 12, 15, 16, 208, 209, 210, 215, 252
Blood 6, 13, 20, 24, 26, 44, 47, 50, 52, 71, 73, 83, 84, 100, 111, 119, 122, 127, 133, 139, 141, 150, 160, 168, 169, 175, 188, 204, 253, 254, 255, 256, 258, 269, 273
Bone 44, 52, 81, 211, 224, 286
Brain 8, 30, 71, 122, 123, 136, 150, 202, 203, 246, 247, 257, 268
Bumps 152, 153, 286
Burn 54, 177, 225, 273, 286

C

Cancer 3, 58, 59, 60, 111, 150, 152, 192, 202, 234, 254, 255, 256, 257, 268, 269, 271, 272, 273, 286
Canine Cognitive Disorder 3, 63, 234, 286
Cardamom 15, 16, 39, 59, 60, 168, 170, 247, 252, 269
Cassia 12, 15, 16, 66, 258, 274
Cat Scratch Fever 50, 114
Cedarwood 123, 124, 165, 166, 224, 226, 227, 230, 238, 253

References

Chemical 9, 12, 13, 33, 38, 54, 57, 58, 59, 60, 69, 103, 122, 131, 152, 160, 167, 177, 252, 253, 254, 257, 271, 272
Chew 65, 66, 80, 86, 163, 177, 198, 258, 286
Cinnamon Bark 16, 271
Cleanser 20, 21, 73, 75, 76, 103, 113, 127, 130, 154, 155, 156, 244, 245
Cleansing Blend 33, 34, 77, 114, 115, 116, 127, 128, 129, 148, 149, 179, 180, 181, 182, 192, 193, 194, 198, 199, 200, 216, 238, 239, 255, 256
Constipation 36, 67, 252, 271, 274, 286
Copaiba 15, 27, 30, 31, 44, 45, 46, 47, 48, 49, 51, 52, 59, 60, 61, 62, 63, 64, 72, 81, 82, 84, 106, 107, 109, 110, 112, 119, 120, 133, 134, 139, 140, 146, 154, 155, 159, 160, 162, 165, 166, 167, 168, 169, 170, 171, 172, 173, 174, 175, 176, 179, 180, 181, 182, 188, 189, 198, 199, 202, 203, 206, 207, 209, 210, 212, 213, 214, 220, 221, 224, 226, 227, 232, 233, 235, 236, 239, 242, 243, 244, 247, 249, 250, 253
Coprophagia 69, 286
Coriander 83
Cushing's Disease 71, 269, 274, 276, 286
Cuts 33, 34, 73, 83, 163, 208, 224, 286
Cypress 16, 30, 31, 123, 124, 133, 134, 168, 170, 216, 224, 226, 227, 232, 233, 234, 235, 236, 237, 253

D

Delivery 150, 184, 187, 286
Dementia 3, 270, 271
Demodex 77, 286
Dental 65, 80, 81, 151, 256, 286
Depression 38, 144, 150, 175, 219, 252, 253, 254, 255, 257
Detoxification 27, 72, 167, 169, 172, 241, 242, 243, 254, 257
Detoxification Blend 27, 72, 167, 169, 172, 242, 243, 254, 257
Diabetes 83, 84, 141, 234, 256, 275, 286
Diarrhea 24, 26, 27, 36, 50, 86, 87, 89, 101, 108, 111, 148, 167, 177, 192, 246, 248, 252, 253, 256, 286
Diet 20, 21, 27, 31, 32, 39, 44, 47, 49, 58, 60, 63, 67, 68, 69, 70, 72, 77, 81, 84, 85, 86, 87, 89, 90, 91, 96, 97, 103, 106, 107, 109, 110, 112, 125, 131, 139, 140, 141, 144, 145, 152, 153, 160, 161, 175, 179, 181, 182, 183, 184, 189, 193, 194, 199, 203, 206, 207, 212, 213, 214, 220, 221, 232, 235, 236, 237, 241, 242, 243, 244, 247, 249
Diuretic 232, 234, 252, 269
Dry Skin 90, 255, 257, 286

E

Ear Cleaner 92, 94, 95, 286
Ear Infection 32, 92, 94, 96, 126, 143, 202, 246, 254
Ear Mites 98, 286
Ears 10, 12, 32, 92, 93, 94, 95, 96, 98, 126, 127, 128, 129, 136, 137, 167, 195, 202, 206, 286
Emotional 8, 9, 30, 65, 86, 87, 100, 102, 121, 122, 123, 150, 257, 258, 269, 286

Essential Oil 1, 2, 3, 7, 8, 9, 10, 11, 12, 13, 14, 15, 16, 18, 19, 27, 30, 39, 44, 45, 46, 48,
    52, 59, 63, 64, 65, 66, 67, 69, 71, 74, 75, 76, 80, 84, 90, 94, 96, 98, 102, 103, 106,
    108, 109, 111, 112, 113, 114, 119, 122, 123, 133, 135, 139, 144, 145, 146, 148,
    150, 152, 160, 164, 165, 175, 179, 180, 192, 195, 197, 198, 200, 202, 205, 212,
    219, 224, 226, 227, 231, 238, 246, 247, 252, 268, 271, 272, 273, 274, 275, 276
Eucalyptus 15, 16, 168, 170, 222, 253, 254

F

Feline Immunodeficiency Virus 58, 108, 268, 286
Fennel 15, 72, 88, 185, 186
First Aid 113, 136, 208, 286
Flea Bomb 114, 115, 117
Fleas 32, 33, 34, 50, 114, 115, 125, 133, 135, 202, 215, 220, 221, 248, 286
Flea & Tick Repellent Shampoo or Spray 117
Frankincense 15, 27, 33, 34, 44, 45, 46, 47, 48, 49, 50, 51, 54, 55, 59, 60, 61, 62, 63, 64,
    72, 74, 75, 76, 96, 97, 106, 107, 109, 110, 112, 113, 133, 134, 136, 137, 138, 139,
    140, 141, 142, 144, 145, 146, 150, 151, 152, 153, 154, 155, 159, 160, 162, 165,
    166, 168, 170, 173, 174, 175, 176, 179, 180, 181, 182, 183, 184, 185, 187, 188,
    189, 192, 193, 194, 195, 196, 198, 199, 202, 203, 206, 207, 209, 210, 212, 213,
    214, 220, 221, 224, 225, 226, 227, 228, 235, 236, 237, 242, 243, 244, 247, 249,
    250, 254, 269, 273
Fungal 8, 108, 111, 192, 195, 244, 255, 256, 273

G

Gastric 119, 286
Geranium 20, 21, 27, 59, 60, 62, 72, 74, 75, 76, 77, 78, 84, 85, 96, 97, 98, 102, 106, 107,
    109, 110, 112, 114, 116, 139, 140, 154, 155, 169, 172, 180, 181, 182, 195, 196,
    200, 220, 221, 232, 233, 234, 235, 236, 237, 242, 243, 254
Ginger 12, 15, 16, 25, 44, 45, 46, 173, 180, 181, 182, 224, 226, 227, 252
Grapefruit 60, 61, 146, 147, 254
Green Cleaning 54, 103, 105, 111, 131, 143, 152, 167, 202, 238
Grief 38, 86, 100, 101, 102, 105, 121, 122, 123, 238, 253, 255, 286
Grooming 32, 47, 60, 105, 108, 111, 121, 125, 131, 139, 198, 286
Grounding Blend 27, 47, 49, 52, 53, 59, 61, 62, 64, 69, 70, 84, 85, 106, 107, 109, 110, 112,
    113, 139, 140, 141, 142, 144, 145, 159, 164, 165, 166, 179, 180, 181, 182, 188,
    189, 202, 203, 206, 207, 209, 210, 213, 214, 224, 226, 227, 238, 239, 247, 254

H

Hairballs 125, 131, 286
Hand Sanitizer 248, 250
Heartworm 133, 135, 286
Heat Stroke 113, 136, 286
Helichrysum 15, 37, 47, 48, 49, 52, 53, 73, 74, 75, 76, 77, 81, 82, 113, 134, 136, 137, 138,
    167, 168, 169, 170, 171, 172, 173, 174, 180, 181, 182, 188, 189, 197, 198, 199,
    200, 201, 202, 203, 209, 210, 220, 221, 224, 225, 226, 227, 228, 231, 242, 243,
    254, 255, 274
Herpes 105, 106, 274
Hyperthyroidism 139, 286

References

Hypoglycemia 141, 202, 286
Hypothyroidism 30, 143, 144, 246, 286

I

Infection 15, 32, 33, 34, 47, 50, 71, 73, 74, 75, 83, 84, 92, 94, 95, 96, 105, 106, 108, 109, 111, 112, 126, 127, 133, 143, 154, 167, 179, 180, 184, 188, 189, 195, 198, 202, 208, 215, 219, 224, 232, 234, 236, 237, 238, 244, 246, 252, 254, 255, 256
Inflammation 36, 44, 52, 81, 94, 101, 108, 119, 154, 160, 175, 180, 188, 198, 208, 209, 224, 232, 234, 235, 244, 258, 275
Insulin 83, 84, 141, 275

J

Juniper Berry 30, 31, 139, 159, 168, 169, 171, 220, 221, 232, 233, 234, 235, 236, 237, 239, 242, 243

K

Kidney 27, 71, 80, 87, 100, 102, 139, 159, 167, 168, 169, 171, 218, 232, 234, 239, 253, 255

L

Labor 184, 185, 187, 286
Lavender 15, 16, 20, 21, 22, 32, 33, 34, 35, 39, 44, 45, 46, 50, 51, 52, 53, 54, 55, 59, 60, 62, 63, 64, 67, 68, 74, 75, 76, 77, 90, 94, 96, 97, 98, 103, 113, 115, 119, 120, 131, 132, 136, 137, 138, 139, 140, 148, 152, 153, 154, 155, 160, 162, 165, 166, 168, 169, 170, 171, 173, 174, 175, 176, 180, 181, 182, 183, 184, 187, 188, 189, 193, 194, 195, 196, 197, 198, 199, 200, 201, 202, 203, 205, 206, 207, 208, 209, 210, 212, 214, 215, 216, 220, 221, 224, 225, 226, 227, 228, 231, 232, 233, 234, 235, 236, 237, 238, 239, 244, 247, 249, 250, 255, 270, 271, 275
Lemon 33, 54, 55, 60, 61, 81, 82, 133, 134, 144, 145, 255
Lemongrass 12, 16, 48, 59, 143, 144, 145, 148, 180, 181, 182, 195, 196, 232, 233, 234, 235, 236, 237, 249, 250, 255
Lethargy 11, 27, 47, 87, 89, 101, 105, 111, 133, 141, 144, 167, 175, 177, 188, 208, 219
leukemia 58
Leukemia 58, 111, 268, 286
Lipoma 146, 152, 286
Litter Box Power 13, 39, 60, 62, 68, 75, 76, 84, 119, 120, 131, 132, 139, 140, 148, 149, 159, 165, 166, 168, 169, 170, 171, 172, 173, 174, 175, 176, 183, 212, 214, 232, 233, 235, 237, 238, 239, 249, 250, 286
Liver 12, 13, 27, 59, 80, 87, 100, 141, 167, 241, 242, 253, 255
Longevity 6, 44, 106, 109, 112, 150, 160, 220, 286
Lumps 152, 153, 286
Lyme 114, 218

M

Magnolia 43, 255
Marjoram 12, 15, 16, 41, 123, 124, 168, 169, 171, 173, 174, 255, 256
Massage Blend 44, 45, 52, 53, 59, 60, 62, 113, 115, 136, 137, 138, 168, 170, 173, 174,

175, 176, 180, 181, 182, 215, 224, 226, 227, 232, 233, 234, 236, 237, 242, 243, 252, 253, 254, 256
Mastitis 154, 286
Melaleuca 12, 256, 268
Melissa 106, 107, 109, 110, 112, 152, 153, 247
Metabolism 84, 271, 275
Mosquito 32, 33, 34, 50, 114, 115, 133, 135, 202, 215, 220, 221, 248, 268, 270, 271
Myrrh 15, 16, 20, 21, 23, 30, 31, 32, 33, 34, 39, 48, 49, 50, 51, 59, 60, 62, 67, 68, 74, 75, 76, 80, 81, 82, 84, 85, 86, 88, 90, 96, 97, 103, 113, 115, 119, 120, 134, 139, 140, 144, 145, 152, 153, 154, 155, 160, 162, 169, 172, 173, 174, 180, 181, 182, 183, 184, 185, 187, 195, 196, 197, 198, 199, 200, 208, 210, 220, 221, 231, 235, 236, 237, 244, 249, 250, 256, 273

N

Nausea 180, 208, 246, 247, 253, 276
Nerve 271, 275
Neurologic 30, 31, 63, 108, 150, 180, 202, 203, 206, 212, 254, 258, 286
New Pet Parents 158, 286
Nutrition 7, 24, 32, 36, 38, 44, 52, 58, 64, 71, 75, 76, 90, 101, 103, 151, 160, 161, 167, 184, 203, 234, 244, 286

O

Obsessive-Compulsive Disorder 66, 131, 163, 286
Oregano 12, 15, 16, 134, 152, 153, 189, 256
Organ Support 27, 83, 87, 133, 139, 141, 167, 218, 225, 232, 234, 286
Outdoor Blend 98, 114, 115, 116, 215, 216, 252, 253, 254, 258

P

Pain 14, 15, 20, 29, 36, 44, 52, 59, 60, 73, 74, 80, 81, 119, 127, 161, 173, 175, 179, 180, 181, 182, 188, 202, 208, 215, 218, 219, 224, 232, 234, 235, 252, 254, 255, 256, 258, 274, 286
Pancreas 83, 175, 286
Pancreatitis 83, 175, 268, 286
Parasite 6, 86, 87, 98, 114, 151, 192, 218, 248, 256
Peppermint 12, 16, 32, 33, 80, 113, 136, 137, 138, 216, 256
Pet Powder 127, 128, 130
Pink Pepper 12, 59, 60, 257
Poison 57, 113, 152, 177, 286
Pre-and Post Operative Care 179, 286
Pregnancy 16, 184, 187, 248, 276, 286
Probiotic 7, 20, 21, 24, 27, 31, 39, 49, 52, 60, 64, 67, 68, 69, 70, 72, 75, 77, 81, 84, 85, 87, 89, 90, 91, 97, 103, 106, 107, 109, 110, 112, 119, 120, 125, 131, 139, 140, 144, 145, 152, 153, 160, 161, 167, 175, 179, 181, 182, 183, 189, 193, 194, 199, 203, 206, 207, 212, 213, 214, 220, 221, 232, 234, 235, 236, 237, 241, 242, 243, 244, 247, 249
Prostate 188, 286
Protective Blend 15, 20, 21, 27, 33, 34, 47, 48, 49, 50, 51, 54, 55, 60, 61, 62, 72, 75, 76, 80, 81, 82, 84, 85, 86, 88, 97, 105, 106, 107, 109, 110, 112, 113, 114, 115, 119,

References

      120, 133, 134, 144, 145, 152, 153, 154, 155, 176, 179, 180, 181, 182, 192, 193, 194, 195, 196, 198, 199, 209, 210, 225, 227, 228, 232, 235, 236, 238, 239, 244, 248, 249, 250, 254, 258
Puppy 29, 65, 66, 69, 154, 158, 184, 186, 187
Pyometra 190, 286

R

Reassuring Blend 27, 67, 68, 69, 70, 86, 87, 88, 123, 124, 159, 165, 179, 180, 181, 182, 206, 207, 209, 210, 212, 238, 239
Renewing Blend 31, 106, 107, 109, 110, 112, 169, 172, 193, 194, 224, 225, 226, 227, 228
Respiratory Blend 50, 51, 136, 137, 167, 170, 192, 193, 194, 225, 226, 227, 228, 252, 254, 255, 256
Respiratory Conditions 101, 105, 150, 167, 192, 225, 252, 253, 286
Restful Blend 24, 27, 31, 41, 52, 53, 54, 55, 60, 61, 63, 64, 67, 68, 69, 70, 72, 75, 84, 85, 86, 87, 88, 106, 107, 109, 110, 112, 113, 123, 131, 132, 141, 142, 154, 155, 159, 164, 165, 166, 176, 179, 180, 181, 182, 184, 187, 193, 194, 202, 203, 206, 207, 209, 210, 212, 213, 214, 238, 239, 247, 253, 255, 258
Ringworm 195, 286
Rosemary 15, 16, 98, 133, 148, 169, 172, 183, 238, 239, 243

S

Salve 20, 21, 23, 54, 55, 56, 77, 79, 103, 104, 113, 154, 155, 156, 180, 181, 182, 195, 196, 197, 198, 199, 200, 224, 225, 228, 231
Sandalwood 59, 60, 62, 90, 91, 152, 257, 270
Scabies 198, 199, 286
Second Hand Smoke 192
Sedative 269
Seizure 15, 71, 108, 136, 141, 143, 177, 202, 203, 286
Shampoo 22, 32, 33, 34, 77, 78, 90, 91, 114, 115, 116, 117, 126, 195, 196, 197, 198, 199, 200, 220, 221, 223
Sleep 63, 121, 167, 271
Snake Bites 208, 286
Sound Sensitivity 211, 286
Spider Bites 32, 33, 34, 215
Spiders 215, 216, 286
Stress 24, 26, 27, 28, 30, 31, 38, 40, 52, 60, 63, 64, 65, 67, 69, 71, 72, 84, 86, 105, 106, 109, 112, 131, 141, 143, 148, 154, 159, 163, 165, 167, 179, 184, 195, 199, 206, 211, 212, 234, 238, 255, 272, 286
Sunburn 198, 199, 201

T

Thyme 12, 16, 48, 59, 106, 107, 109, 110, 112, 114, 116, 188, 189, 208, 210, 220, 221, 257
Tick 32, 33, 34, 50, 114, 116, 125, 133, 135, 202, 215, 218, 219, 220, 221, 248, 254, 268, 272, 275, 286
Trauma 44, 202, 208, 224, 227, 228, 246, 247, 286
Tumor 8, 30, 59, 71, 72, 146, 202, 246, 269
Turmeric 173, 174

U

Urinary 63, 83, 188, 189, 232, 234, 238, 244, 252, 253, 286
Urinating Outside of the Litter Box 238, 286
Urine 26, 63, 111, 188, 232, 234, 238, 240

V

Vaccine 241, 286
Vaccine Detoxification 241
Vaginitis 244, 286
Vestibular Disease 202, 246, 286
Vetiver 16, 180, 181, 182, 212, 213, 214, 258
Vomiting 13, 24, 26, 27, 36, 38, 50, 57, 86, 87, 89, 108, 111, 148, 167, 175, 177, 188, 192, 246, 247, 248, 256, 276, 286

W

Wintergreen 15, 16
Worms 133, 248, 286
Wound 20, 21, 32, 47, 73, 74, 75, 76, 108, 163, 180, 181, 182, 209, 224, 226, 227, 253, 256, 268, 276

Y

Ylang Ylang 72, 84, 133, 134, 167, 168, 169, 170, 171, 188, 189, 232, 233, 235, 237, 239, 258, 259

"Until one has loved an animal, a part of one's soul remains unawakened."

Anatole France

References

Connect with Dr. Mia Frezzo and Jan Jeremias at www.spoilyourpeteo.com

TABLE OF AILMENTS

Ailments		Page
Abscesses		20
Acid Reflux		24
Addison's Disease		26
Aggressive Behavior		28
Allergies		32
Anal Glands		36
Anorexia/Loss of Appetite		38
Anxiety and Stress		40
Arthritis		44
Autoimmune Disorders		47
Bartonella		50
Broken Bones/Bone Pain		52
Burns		54
Cancer		58
Canine Cognitive Disorder		63
Chewing		65
Constipation		67
Coprophagia		69
Cushing's Disease		71
Cuts and Scrapes		73
Demodex/Mange		77
Dental Care		80
Diabetes		83
Diarrhea and Vomiting		86
Dry Skin		90
Ear Cleaning		92
Ear Infections		96
Ear Mites		98
Emotions and Organs		100
Feline Acne		103
Feline Herpesvirus (FVH-1)		105
Feline Immunodeficiency Virus		108
Feline Leukemia Virus		111
First Aid for Pets		113
Fleas/Ticks/Mosquitos		114
Gastric Ulcers		119
Grief and Loss		121
Grooming/Basic Pet Care		125
Hair Balls		131
Heartworm Disease		133
Heat Stroke		136

Ailments		Page
Hyperthyroidism		139
Hypoglycemia		141
Hypothyroidism		143
Lipomas/Fatty Tumors		146
Litter Box Power		148
Longevity		150
Lumps and Bumps		152
Mastitis		154
New Pet Parents/Introducing A New Pet		158
Nutrition		160
Obsessive-Compulsive Disorder (OCD)		163
Organ Support		167
Pain		173
Pancreatitis		175
Poisoning		177
Preoperative/Post-operative Care		179
Pregnancy, Labor and Delivery		184
Prostatic Disease		188
Pyometra (Uterine Infection)		190
Respiratory Conditions		192
Ringworm		195
Scabies		198
Seizures and Neurologic Conditions		202
Separation Anxiety		204
Snakebite		208
Sound Sensitivity		211
Spider Bite		215
Tick-Borne Diseases		218
Trauma		224
Urinary Blockage		232
Urinary Conditions		234
Urinating Outside of Litter Box		238
Vaccination Detoxification		241
Vaginitis		244
Vestibular Disease		246
Worms/Intestinal Parasites		248

KEY   For Dogs: For Cats: For Dogs & Cats: